TOWER AIR FRYER COOKBOOK FOR BEGINNERS

QUICK AND EASY BUDGET FRIENDLY

AIR FRYER RECIPES

ROY FABELA

CONTENTS

INTRODUCTION **7**

Getting to Know Your Tower Air Fryer 7

The Benefits You'll Gain from Your Tower Air Fryer 7

How You Should Start with Your Tower Air Fryer 8

Better to Care for Your Tower Air Fryer 9

VEGETABLE SIDE DISHES RECIPES **10**

Parmesan Asparagus 10

Hush Puppies 11

Broccoli Tots 12

Shoestring Butternut Squash Fries 13

Steak Fries 14

Mini Hasselback Potatoes 15

Perfect French Fries 16

Cheesy Potato Pot 17

Asparagus Fries 18

Fried Eggplant Balls 19

POULTRY RECIPES **20**

Cornish Hens With Honey-lime Glaze 20

Chicken Tikka 21

Chicken Adobo 22

Buffalo Egg Rolls 23

Chicken Hand Pies 24

Southern-fried Chicken Livers 25

Chicken Chimichangas 26

Chicken Cordon Bleu 27

Coconut Curry Chicken With Coconut Rice 28

Lemon Sage Roast Chicken 29

Teriyaki Chicken Legs 30

Tandoori Chicken Legs 31

BEEF, PORK & LAMB RECIPES **32**
Wasabi-coated Pork Loin Chops 32
Crispy Ham And Eggs 33
Bacon Wrapped Filets Mignons 34
Apple Cornbread Stuffed Pork Loin With Apple Gravy 35
Sloppy Joes 36
Pepperoni Pockets 37
Chicken-fried Steak 38
Chicken Fried Steak 39
Pork & Beef Egg Rolls 40
California Burritos 41
Cinnamon-stick Kofta Skewers 42
Honey Mesquite Pork Chops 43

APPETIZERS AND SNACKS **44**
Eggs In Avocado Halves 44
Fried Pickles 45
Classic Potato Chips 46
Spanakopita Spinach, Feta And Pine Nut Phyllo Bites 47
Country Wings 48
Sausage And Cheese Rolls 49
Fried Goat Cheese 50
Smoked Salmon Puffs 51
Mozzarella En Carrozza With Puttanesca Sauce 52
Potato Chips With Sour Cream And Onion Dip 53
Cuban Sliders 54
Zucchini Fritters 55

BREAD AND BREAKFAST **56**
Quesadillas 56
Parmesan Garlic Naan 57
Western Omelet 58
Green Onion Pancakes 59
Tuscan Toast 60
Farmers Market Quiche 61

Broccoli Cornbread 62
Coffee Cake 63
Mini Pita Breads 64
Garlic Bread Knots 65
Walnut Pancake 66
Hush Puffins 67

VEGETARIANS RECIPES 68

Basic Fried Tofu 68
Falafels 69
Roasted Vegetable Thai Green Curry 70
Mushroom And Fried Onion Quesadilla 71
Tacos 72
Broccoli Cheddar Stuffed Potatoes 73
Spicy Vegetable And Tofu Shake Fry 74
Curried Potato, Cauliflower And Pea Turnovers 75
Asparagus, Mushroom And Cheese Soufflés 77
Pizza Portobello Mushrooms 78
Eggplant Parmesan 79

DESSERTS AND SWEETS 80

Blueberry Cheesecake Tartlets 80
Puff Pastry Apples 81
Oreo-coated Peanut Butter Cups 82
Maple Cinnamon Cheesecake 83
Cherry Hand Pies 84
Donut Holes 85
Giant Oatmeal–peanut Butter Cookie 86
Custard 87
Sea-salted Caramel Cookie Cups 88
Blueberry Crisp 89
S'mores Pockets 90
Sweet Potato Pie Rolls 91

FISH AND SEAFOOD RECIPES 92

Bacon-wrapped Scallops ... 92
Italian Tuna Roast ... 93
Stuffed Shrimp ... 94
Tuna Nuggets In Hoisin Sauce ... 95
Five Spice Red Snapper With Green Onions And Orange Salsa ... 96
Lemon-roasted Salmon Fillets ... 97
Shrimp Teriyaki ... 98
Shrimp "scampi" ... 99
Shrimp Patties ... 100
Salmon Puttanesca En Papillotte With Zucchini ... 101

SANDWICHES AND BURGERS RECIPES ... 102

Sausage And Pepper Heros ... 102
Best-ever Roast Beef Sandwiches ... 103
Chili Cheese Dogs ... 104
Perfect Burgers ... 105
Thai-style Pork Sliders ... 106
Crunchy Falafel Balls ... 107
Lamb Burgers ... 108
Thanksgiving Turkey Sandwiches ... 109
Chicken Spiedies ... 110

INTRODUCTION

Getting to Know Your Tower Air Fryer

An air fryer is actually a lot like a countertop convection oven. It's a small electric appliance with a heating element and a fan that blows air around in a cooking chamber. However, in an air fryer, the air is swirled very quickly in a circular fashion — so it does a better job of reaching all of the surfaces of the food and creating a crisp crust. Plus, the food itself sits in a perforated basket which increases its contact with the hot moving air. Another thing that makes a big difference? The fact that there's not much space between the walls of the chamber, and the basket intensifies the heat.

The Benefits You'll Gain from Your Tower Air Fryer

1. WEIGHT LOSS POTENTIAL

If you're driven to lose weight, you can do so by slowly making changes in your eating and cooking habits. Research shows that cooking your food with an air fryer (versus a deep fryer) can be healthier, thus potentially reducing your caloric intake and contributing to weight loss. Considering that fried food can factor into obesity, weight loss potential is among the most compelling draws of the air fryer.

Additionally, the need for significantly less oil helps consumers be mindful of their cholesterol levels. Since air fryers only require a few drops of oil, it's easier to enjoy comfort food faves, like French fries, while keeping minimal saturated fat content.

2. FASTER FOOD PREP

Air fryers are very time-efficient. Foods including chicken, fish, potatoes, and vegetables all cook quickly in an air fryer. This ability is attributed to technology that allows the air fryer to blow hot air evenly within the device.

3. EASIER CLEAN UP

Not only will you exert less effort and spend less time cooking with an air fryer, but you'll also have a much easier time cleaning up. Many of its parts are designed to be wiped off with a damp cloth or washed in the sink with soap. Some air fryers even have parts that are dishwasher-safe. Overall, they're much easier to clean and maintain than larger cooking gadgets.

4. MORE SPACE, LESS STINK

Air fryers also take up less space in the kitchen, which is especially beneficial if you have a smaller space. Another bonus: An air fryer won't leave your house with lingering fried food smells for hours after cooking.

5. GREAT FOR PICKY VEGETABLE EATERS

Are you and your loved ones picky vegetable eaters? Air frying is a great way to crisp up vegetables and make them tastier. Many people enjoy the texture of vegetables such as cauliflower, broccoli, or Brussels sprouts better once they've been air fried. There are also a myriad of online recipes that give options for breading vegetables to cook in the air fryer. Some even incorporate lighter options like rice- or chickpea-based crumbs.

How You Should Start with Your Tower Air Fryer

1. PREPARATION OF THE FOOD

To prevent the food from sticking to the fryer basket, add bare minimum oil. Let space between the food to allow the hot air to pass through and cook from all sides. Use an aluminum foil paper as a separator. If you are using marinated or oily ingredients then pat them dry. This will avoid any splattering or excess smoke. Remove any oil / fat from the bottom of the fryer.

2. PREPARATION OF THE Tower AIR FRYER

Plug in the fryer and preheat it for about 5 minutes. Ensure that your air fryer is hot enough.

Place the food items inside and avoid overcrowding. Air must be able to circulate through all the sides of each food item to properly cook it. If you are cooking pre-made foods, you can change the initial oven temperature by 70 degrees and cut the cooking time in half.

3. COOKING IN THE Tower AIR FRYER

While cooking small food items like chicken wings or fries, try to shake the fryer around a couple of times. Also try rotating the food items every five minutes to guarantee an all-rounded fry. If you are cooking high fat food, you will find that it releases fat in the base of the fryer. You would need to remove this fat after cooking.

Better to Care for Your Tower Air Fryer

1. UNPLUG AND ALLOW TO COOL

After every use, unplug the air fryer from the wall outlet and allow the unit to cool completely before cleaning any component.

Wash Removable Components

Once the unit is cool, remove the crisper plate or tray and basket. These can be hand washed with dish-washing liquid and hot water or placed in the dishwasher. Always check the user guide that came with the air fryer to make sure these components are dishwasher-safe. Most manufacturers recommend hand-washing the baskets to extend their life.

2. DRY THE COMPONENTS

If you are handwashing or stop the dishwasher before the drying cycle, use a lint-free microfiber cloth to dry the crisper plate and basket. Never put damp components back into the base unit.

Wipe Down the Base Unit

Dampen a non-abrasive sponge with warm water and add a drop of dish-washing liquid. With the unit unplugged and with the basket, plates or trays removed, use the sponge to wipe out the entire interior opening. Use a microfiber cloth to thoroughly dry the area.

Rinse out the sponge and use it to wipe down the exterior of the appliance including the control panel.

3. DO A DEEP CLEAN

After several uses, check the heating element for grease splatters or food particles. Use a damp non-abrasive sponge to wipe it clean.

If the air fryer develops a bad odor, there are food splatters somewhere in the interior. In a small bowl, mix one tablespoon of water with two tablespoons of baking soda to make a paste. Dip a dampened sponge in the paste to clean the interior. You may also need to use a small soft-bristled brush like a bottle brush or an old toothbrush dipped in the solution to get into all of the corners. Rinse with a sponge dipped in clean water and dry thoroughly with a microfiber cloth before reinserting the basket and plates and plugging the unit into a wall outlet.

VEGETABLE SIDE DISHES RECIPES

Parmesan Asparagus

Servings: 2

Cooking Time: 5 Minutes

Ingredients:

- 1 bunch asparagus, stems trimmed
- 1 teaspoon olive oil
- salt and freshly ground black pepper
- ¼ cup coarsely grated Parmesan cheese
- ½ lemon

Directions:

1. Preheat the air fryer to 400°F.
2. Toss the asparagus with the oil and season with salt and freshly ground black pepper.
3. Transfer the asparagus to the air fryer basket and air-fry at 400°F for 5 minutes, shaking the basket to turn the asparagus once or twice during the cooking process.
4. When the asparagus is cooked to your liking, sprinkle the asparagus generously with the Parmesan cheese and close the air fryer drawer again. Let the asparagus sit for 1 minute in the turned-off air fryer. Then, remove the asparagus, transfer it to a serving dish and finish with a grind of black pepper and a squeeze of lemon juice.

Hush Puppies

Servings: 8

Cooking Time: 11 Minutes

Ingredients:

- ½ cup Whole or low-fat milk (not fat-free)
- 1½ tablespoons Butter
- ½ cup plus 1 tablespoon, plus more All-purpose flour
- ½ cup plus 1 tablespoon Yellow cornmeal
- 2 teaspoons Granulated white sugar
- 2 teaspoons Baking powder
- ¾ teaspoon Baking soda
- ¾ teaspoon Table salt
- ¼ teaspoon Onion powder
- 3 tablespoons (or 1 medium egg, well beaten) Pasteurized egg substitute, such as Egg Beaters
- Vegetable oil spray

Directions:

1. Heat the milk and butter in a small saucepan set over medium heat just until the butter melts and the milk is steamy. Do not simmer or boil.
2. Meanwhile, whisk the flour, cornmeal, sugar, baking powder, baking soda, salt, and onion powder in a large bowl until the mixture is a uniform color.
3. Stir the hot milk mixture into the flour mixture to form a dough. Set aside to cool for 5 minutes.
4. Mix the egg substitute or egg into the dough to make a thick, smooth batter. Cover and refrigerate for at least 1 hour or up to 4 hours.
5. Preheat the air fryer to 350°F .
6. Lightly flour your clean, dry hands. Roll 2 tablespoons of the batter into a ball between your floured palms. Set aside, flour your hands again if necessary, and continue making more balls with the remaining batter.
7. Coat the balls all over with the vegetable oil spray. Line the machine's basket (or basket attachment) with a piece of parchment paper. Set the balls on the parchment paper with as much air space between them as possible. Air-fry for 9 minutes, or until lightly browned and set.
8. Use kitchen tongs to gently transfer the hush puppies to a wire rack. Cool for at least 5 minutes before serving. Or cool to room temperature, about 45 minutes, and store in a sealed container at room temperature for up to 2 days. To crisp the hush puppies again, put them in a 350°F air fryer for 2 minutes. (There's no need for parchment paper in the machine during reheating.)

Broccoli Tots

Servings: 24

Cooking Time: 10 Minutes

Ingredients:

- 2 cups broccoli florets (about ½ pound broccoli crowns)
- 1 egg, beaten
- ⅛ teaspoon onion powder
- ¼ teaspoon salt
- ⅛ teaspoon pepper
- 2 tablespoons grated Parmesan cheese
- ¼ cup panko breadcrumbs
- oil for misting

Directions:

1. Steam broccoli for 2minutes. Rinse in cold water, drain well, and chop finely.
2. In a large bowl, mix broccoli with all other ingredients except the oil.
3. Scoop out small portions of mixture and shape into 24 tots. Lay them on a cookie sheet or wax paper as you work.
4. Spray tots with oil and place in air fryer basket in single layer.
5. Cook at 390°F for 5minutes. Shake basket and spray with oil again. Cook 5minutes longer or until browned and crispy.

Shoestring Butternut Squash Fries

Servings: 3

Cooking Time: 16 Minutes

Ingredients:

- 1 pound 2 ounces Spiralized butternut squash strands
- Vegetable oil spray
- To taste Coarse sea salt or kosher salt

Directions:

1. Preheat the air fryer to 375°F .
2. Place the spiralized squash in a big bowl. Coat the strands with vegetable oil spray, toss well, coat again, and toss several times to make sure all the strands have been oiled.
3. When the machine is at temperature, pour the strands into the basket and spread them out into as even a layer as possible. Air-fry for 16 minutes, tossing and rearranging the strands every 4 minutes, or until they're lightly browned and crisp.
4. Pour the contents of the basket into a serving bowl, add salt to taste, and toss well before serving hot.

Steak Fries

Servings: 4

Cooking Time: 20 Minutes

Ingredients:

- 2 russet potatoes, scrubbed and cut into wedges lengthwise
- 1 tablespoon olive oil
- 2 teaspoons seasoning salt (recipe below)

Directions:

1. Preheat the air fryer to 400°F.
2. Toss the potatoes with the olive oil and the seasoning salt.
3. Air-fry for 20 minutes (depending on the size of the wedges), turning the potatoes over gently a few times throughout the cooking process to brown and cook them evenly.

Mini Hasselback Potatoes

Servings: 4

Cooking Time: 25 Minutes

Ingredients:

- 1½ pounds baby Yukon Gold potatoes (about 10)
- 5 tablespoons butter, cut into very thin slices
- salt and freshly ground black pepper
- 1 tablespoon vegetable oil
- ¼ cup grated Parmesan cheese (optional)
- chopped fresh parsley or chives

Directions:

1. Preheat the air fryer to 400°F.
2. Make six to eight deep vertical slits across the top of each potato about three quarters of the way down. Make sure the slits are deep enough to allow the slices to spread apart a little, but don't cut all the way through the potato. Place a thin slice of butter between each of the slices and season generously with salt and pepper.
3. Transfer the potatoes to the air fryer basket. Pack them in next to each other. It's alright if some of the potatoes sit on top or rest on another potato. Air-fry for 20 minutes.
4. Spray or brush the potatoes with a little vegetable oil and sprinkle the Parmesan cheese on top. Air-fry for an additional 5 minutes. Garnish with chopped parsley or chives and serve hot.

Perfect French Fries

Servings: 3

Cooking Time: 37 Minutes

Ingredients:

- 1 pound Large russet potato(es)
- Vegetable oil or olive oil spray
- ½ teaspoon Table salt

Directions:

1. Cut each potato lengthwise into ¼-inch-thick slices. Cut each of these lengthwise into ¼-inch-thick matchsticks.
2. Set the potato matchsticks in a big bowl of cool water and soak for 5 minutes. Drain in a colander set in the sink, then spread the matchsticks out on paper towels and dry them very well.
3. Preheat the air fryer to 225°F (or 230°F, if that's the closest setting).
4. When the machine is at temperature, arrange the matchsticks in an even layer (if overlapping but not compact) in the basket. Air-fry for 20 minutes, tossing and rearranging the fries twice.
5. Pour the contents of the basket into a big bowl. Increase the air fryer's temperature to 325°F (or 330°F, if that's the closest setting).
6. Generously coat the fries with vegetable or olive oil spray. Toss well, then coat them again to make sure they're covered on all sides, tossing (and maybe spraying) a couple of times to make sure.
7. When the machine is at temperature, pour the fries into the basket and air-fry for 12 minutes, tossing and rearranging the fries at least twice.
8. Increase the machine's temperature to 375°F (or 380°F or 390°F, if one of these is the closest setting). Air-fry for 5 minutes more (from the moment you raise the temperature), tossing and rearranging the fries at least twice to keep them from burning and to make sure they all get an even measure of the heat, until brown and crisp.
9. Pour the contents of the basket into a serving bowl. Toss the fries with the salt and serve hot.

Cheesy Potato Pot

Servings: 4

Cooking Time: 13 Minutes

Ingredients:

- 3 cups cubed red potatoes (unpeeled, cut into ½-inch cubes)
- ½ teaspoon garlic powder
- salt and pepper
- 1 tablespoon oil
- chopped chives for garnish (optional)
- Sauce
- 2 tablespoons milk
- 1 tablespoon butter
- 2 ounces sharp Cheddar cheese, grated
- 1 tablespoon sour cream

Directions:

1. Place potato cubes in large bowl and sprinkle with garlic, salt, and pepper. Add oil and stir to coat well.
2. Cook at 390°F for 13 minutes or until potatoes are tender. Stir every 4 or 5minutes during cooking time.
3. While potatoes are cooking, combine milk and butter in a small saucepan. Warm over medium-low heat to melt butter. Add cheese and stir until it melts. The melted cheese will remain separated from the milk mixture. Remove from heat until potatoes are done.
4. When ready to serve, add sour cream to cheese mixture and stir over medium-low heat just until warmed. Place cooked potatoes in serving bowl. Pour sauce over potatoes and stir to combine.
5. Garnish with chives if desired.

Asparagus Fries

Servings: 4

Cooking Time: 5 Minutes Per Batch

Ingredients:

- 12 ounces fresh asparagus spears with tough ends trimmed off
- 2 egg whites
- ¼ cup water
- ¾ cup panko breadcrumbs
- ¼ cup grated Parmesan cheese, plus 2 tablespoons
- ¼ teaspoon salt
- oil for misting or cooking spray

Directions:

1. Preheat air fryer to 390°F.
2. In a shallow dish, beat egg whites and water until slightly foamy.
3. In another shallow dish, combine panko, Parmesan, and salt.
4. Dip asparagus spears in egg, then roll in crumbs. Spray with oil or cooking spray.
5. Place a layer of asparagus in air fryer basket, leaving just a little space in between each spear. Stack another layer on top, crosswise. Cook at 390°F for 5 minutes, until crispy and golden brown.
6. Repeat to cook remaining asparagus.

Fried Eggplant Balls

Servings: 4

Cooking Time: 40 Minutes

Ingredients:

- 1 medium eggplant (about 1 pound)
- olive oil
- salt and freshly ground black pepper
- 1 cup grated Parmesan cheese
- 2 cups fresh breadcrumbs
- 2 tablespoons chopped fresh parsley
- 2 tablespoons chopped fresh basil
- 1 clove garlic, minced
- 1 egg, lightly beaten
- ½ cup fine dried breadcrumbs

Directions:

1. Preheat the air fryer to 400°F.
2. Quarter the eggplant by cutting it in half both lengthwise and horizontally. Make a few slashes in the flesh of the eggplant but not through the skin. Brush the cut surface of the eggplant generously with olive oil and transfer to the air fryer basket, cut side up. Air-fry for 10 minutes. Turn the eggplant quarters cut side down and air-fry for another 15 minutes or until the eggplant is soft all the way through. You may need to rotate the pieces in the air fryer so that they cook evenly. Transfer the eggplant to a cutting board to cool.
3. Place the Parmesan cheese, the fresh breadcrumbs, fresh herbs, garlic and egg in a food processor. Scoop the flesh out of the eggplant, discarding the skin and any pieces that are tough. You should have about 1 to 1½ cups of eggplant. Add the eggplant to the food processor and process everything together until smooth. Season with salt and pepper. Refrigerate the mixture for at least 30 minutes.
4. Place the dried breadcrumbs into a shallow dish or onto a plate. Scoop heaping tablespoons of the eggplant mixture into the dried breadcrumbs. Roll the dollops of eggplant in the breadcrumbs and then shape into small balls. You should have 16 to 18 eggplant balls at the end. Refrigerate until you are ready to air-fry.
5. Preheat the air fryer to 350°F.
6. Spray the eggplant balls and the air fryer basket with olive oil. Air-fry the eggplant balls for 15 minutes, rotating the balls during the cooking process to brown evenly.

POULTRY RECIPES

Cornish Hens With Honey-lime Glaze

Servings: 2

Cooking Time: 30 Minutes

Ingredients:

- 1 Cornish game hen (1½–2 pounds)
- 1 tablespoon honey
- 1 tablespoon lime juice
- 1 teaspoon poultry seasoning
- salt and pepper
- cooking spray

Directions:

1. To split the hen into halves, cut through breast bone and down one side of the backbone.
2. Mix the honey, lime juice, and poultry seasoning together and brush or rub onto all sides of the hen. Season to taste with salt and pepper.
3. Spray air fryer basket with cooking spray and place hen halves in the basket, skin-side down.
4. Cook at 330°F for 30 minutes. Hen will be done when juices run clear when pierced at leg joint with a fork. Let hen rest for 5 to 10minutes before cutting.

Chicken Tikka

Servings: 4

Cooking Time: 15 Minutes

Ingredients:

- ¼ cup plain Greek yogurt
- 1 clove garlic, minced
- 1 tablespoon ketchup
- 1 tablespoon extra-virgin olive oil
- 1 tablespoon lemon juice
- ½ teaspoon salt
- ½ teaspoon ground cumin
- ½ teaspoon paprika
- ¼ teaspoon ground cinnamon
- ½ teaspoon ground black pepper
- ½ teaspoon cayenne pepper
- 1 pound boneless, skinless chicken thighs

Directions:

1. In a large bowl, stir together the yogurt, garlic, ketchup, olive oil, lemon juice, salt, cumin, paprika, cinnamon, black pepper, and cayenne pepper until combined.
2. Add the chicken thighs to the bow and fold the yogurt-spice mixture over the chicken thighs until they're covered with the marinade. Cover with plastic wrap and place in the refrigerator for 30 minutes.
3. When ready to cook the chicken, remove from the refrigerator and preheat the air fryer to 370°F.
4. Liberally spray the air fryer basket with olive oil mist. Place the chicken thighs into the air fryer basket, leaving space between the thighs to turn.
5. Cook for 10 minutes, turn the chicken thighs, and cook another 5 minutes (or until the internal temperature reaches 165°F).
6. Remove the chicken from the air fryer and serve warm with desired sides.

Chicken Adobo

Servings: 6

Cooking Time: 12 Minutes

Ingredients:

- 6 boneless chicken thighs
- ¼ cup soy sauce or tamari
- ½ cup rice wine vinegar
- 4 cloves garlic, minced
- ⅛ teaspoon crushed red pepper flakes
- ½ teaspoon black pepper

Directions:

1. Place the chicken thighs into a resealable plastic bag with the soy sauce or tamari, the rice wine vinegar, the garlic, and the crushed red pepper flakes. Seal the bag and let the chicken marinate at least 1 hour in the refrigerator.
2. Preheat the air fryer to 400°F.
3. Drain the chicken and pat dry with a paper towel. Season the chicken with black pepper and liberally spray with cooking spray.
4. Place the chicken in the air fryer basket and cook for 9 minutes, turn over at 9 minutes and check for an internal temperature of 165°F, and cook another 3 minutes.

Buffalo Egg Rolls

Servings: 8

Cooking Time: 9 Minutes Per Batch

Ingredients:

- 1 teaspoon water
- 1 tablespoon cornstarch
- 1 egg
- 2½ cups cooked chicken, diced or shredded (see opposite page)
- ⅓ cup chopped green onion
- ⅓ cup diced celery
- ⅓ cup buffalo wing sauce
- 8 egg roll wraps
- oil for misting or cooking spray
- Blue Cheese Dip
- 3 ounces cream cheese, softened
- ⅓ cup blue cheese, crumbled
- 1 teaspoon Worcestershire sauce
- ¼ teaspoon garlic powder
- ¼ cup buttermilk (or sour cream)

Directions:

1. Mix water and cornstarch in a small bowl until dissolved. Add egg, beat well, and set aside.
2. In a medium size bowl, mix together chicken, green onion, celery, and buffalo wing sauce.
3. Divide chicken mixture evenly among 8 egg roll wraps, spooning ½ inch from one edge.
4. Moisten all edges of each wrap with beaten egg wash.
5. Fold the short ends over filling, then roll up tightly and press to seal edges.
6. Brush outside of wraps with egg wash, then spritz with oil or cooking spray.
7. Place 4 egg rolls in air fryer basket.
8. Cook at 390°F for 9minutes or until outside is brown and crispy.
9. While the rolls are cooking, prepare the Blue Cheese Dip. With a fork, mash together cream cheese and blue cheese.
10. Stir in remaining ingredients.
11. Dip should be just thick enough to slightly cling to egg rolls. If too thick, stir in buttermilk or milk 1 tablespoon at a time until you reach the desired consistency.
12. Cook remaining 4 egg rolls as in steps 7 and 8.
13. Serve while hot with Blue Cheese Dip, more buffalo wing sauce, or both.

Chicken Hand Pies

Servings: 8

Cooking Time: 10 Minutes Per Batch

Ingredients:

- ¾ cup chicken broth
- ¾ cup frozen mixed peas and carrots
- 1 cup cooked chicken, chopped
- 1 tablespoon cornstarch
- 1 tablespoon milk
- salt and pepper
- 1 8-count can organic flaky biscuits
- oil for misting or cooking spray

Directions:

1. In a medium saucepan, bring chicken broth to a boil. Stir in the frozen peas and carrots and cook for 5minutes over medium heat. Stir in chicken.
2. Mix the cornstarch into the milk until it dissolves. Stir it into the simmering chicken broth mixture and cook just until thickened.
3. Remove from heat, add salt and pepper to taste, and let cool slightly.
4. Lay biscuits out on wax paper. Peel each biscuit apart in the middle to make 2 rounds so you have 16 rounds total. Using your hands or a rolling pin, flatten each biscuit round slightly to make it larger and thinner.
5. Divide chicken filling among 8 of the biscuit rounds. Place remaining biscuit rounds on top and press edges all around. Use the tines of a fork to crimp biscuit edges and make sure they are sealed well.
6. Spray both sides lightly with oil or cooking spray.
7. Cook in a single layer, 4 at a time, at 330°F for 10minutes or until biscuit dough is cooked through and golden brown.

Southern-fried Chicken Livers

Servings: 4

Cooking Time: 12 Minutes

Ingredients:

- 2 eggs
- 2 tablespoons water
- ¾ cup flour
- 1½ cups panko breadcrumbs
- ½ cup plain breadcrumbs
- 1 teaspoon salt
- ½ teaspoon black pepper
- 20 ounces chicken livers, salted to taste
- oil for misting or cooking spray

Directions:

1. Beat together eggs and water in a shallow dish. Place the flour in a separate shallow dish.
2. In the bowl of a food processor, combine the panko, plain breadcrumbs, salt, and pepper. Process until well mixed and panko crumbs are finely crushed. Place crumbs in a third shallow dish.
3. Dip livers in flour, then egg wash, and then roll in panko mixture to coat well with crumbs.
4. Spray both sides of livers with oil or cooking spray. Cooking in two batches, place livers in air fryer basket in single layer.
5. Cook at 390°F for 7minutes. Spray livers, turn over, and spray again. Cook for 5 more minutes, until done inside and coating is golden brown.
6. Repeat to cook remaining livers.

Chicken Chimichangas

Servings: 4

Cooking Time: 10 Minutes

Ingredients:

- 2 cups cooked chicken, shredded
- 2 tablespoons chopped green chiles
- ½ teaspoon oregano
- ½ teaspoon cumin
- ½ teaspoon onion powder
- ¼ teaspoon garlic powder
- salt and pepper
- 8 flour tortillas (6- or 7-inch diameter)
- oil for misting or cooking spray
- Chimichanga Sauce
- 2 tablespoons butter
- 2 tablespoons flour
- 1 cup chicken broth
- ¼ cup light sour cream
- ¼ teaspoon salt
- 2 ounces Pepper Jack or Monterey Jack cheese, shredded

Directions:

1. Make the sauce by melting butter in a saucepan over medium-low heat. Stir in flour until smooth and slightly bubbly. Gradually add broth, stirring constantly until smooth. Cook and stir 1 minute, until the mixture slightly thickens. Remove from heat and stir in sour cream and salt. Set aside.
2. In a medium bowl, mix together the chicken, chiles, oregano, cumin, onion powder, garlic, salt, and pepper. Stir in 3 to 4 tablespoons of the sauce, using just enough to make the filling moist but not soupy.
3. Divide filling among the 8 tortillas. Place filling down the center of tortilla, stopping about 1 inch from edges. Fold one side of tortilla over filling, fold the two sides in, and then roll up. Mist all sides with oil or cooking spray.
4. Place chimichangas in air fryer basket seam side down. To fit more into the basket, you can stand them on their sides with the seams against the sides of the basket.
5. Cook at 360°F for 10 minutes or until heated through and crispy brown outside.
6. Add the shredded cheese to the remaining sauce. Stir over low heat, warming just until the cheese melts. Don't boil or sour cream may curdle.
7. Drizzle the sauce over the chimichangas.

Chicken Cordon Bleu

Servings: 2

Cooking Time: 16 Minutes

Ingredients:

- 2 boneless, skinless chicken breasts
- ¼ teaspoon salt
- 2 teaspoons Dijon mustard
- 2 ounces deli ham
- 2 ounces Swiss, fontina, or Gruyère cheese
- ⅓ cup all-purpose flour
- 1 egg
- ½ cup breadcrumbs

Directions:

1. Pat the chicken breasts with a paper towel. Season the chicken with the salt. Pound the chicken breasts to 1½ inches thick. Create a pouch by slicing the side of each chicken breast. Spread 1 teaspoon Dijon mustard inside the pouch of each chicken breast. Wrap a 1-ounce slice of ham around a 1-ounce slice of cheese and place into the pouch. Repeat with the remaining ham and cheese.
2. In a medium bowl, place the flour.
3. In a second bowl, whisk the egg.
4. In a third bowl, place the breadcrumbs.
5. Dredge the chicken in the flour and shake off the excess. Next, dip the chicken into the egg and then in the breadcrumbs. Set the chicken on a plate and repeat with the remaining chicken piece.
6. Preheat the air fryer to 360°F.
7. Place the chicken in the air fryer basket and spray liberally with cooking spray. Cook for 8 minutes, turn the chicken breasts over, and liberally spray with cooking spray again; cook another 6 minutes. Once golden brown, check for an internal temperature of 165°F.

Coconut Curry Chicken With Coconut Rice

Servings: 4

Cooking Time: 56 Minutes

Ingredients:

- 1 (14-ounce) can coconut milk
- 2 tablespoons green or red curry paste
- zest and juice of one lime
- 1 clove garlic, minced
- 1 tablespoon grated fresh ginger
- 1 teaspoon ground cumin
- 1 (3- to 4-pound) chicken, cut into 8 pieces
- vegetable or olive oil
- salt and freshly ground black pepper
- fresh cilantro leaves
- For the rice:
- 1 cup basmati or jasmine rice
- 1 cup water
- 1 cup coconut milk
- ½ teaspoon salt
- freshly ground black pepper

Directions:

1. Make the marinade by combining the coconut milk, curry paste, lime zest and juice, garlic, ginger and cumin. Coat the chicken on all sides with the marinade and marinate the chicken for 1 hour to overnight in the refrigerator.
2. Preheat the air fryer to 380°F.
3. Brush the bottom of the air fryer basket with oil. Transfer the chicken thighs and drumsticks from the marinade to the air fryer basket, letting most of the marinade drip off. Season to taste with salt and freshly ground black pepper.
4. Air-fry the chicken drumsticks and thighs at 380°F for 12 minutes. Flip the chicken over and continue to air-fry for another 12 minutes. Set aside and air-fry the chicken breast pieces at 380°F for 15 minutes. Turn the chicken breast pieces over and air-fry for another 12 minutes. Return the chicken thighs and drumsticks to the air fryer and air-fry for an additional 5 minutes.
5. While the chicken is cooking, make the coconut rice. Rinse the rice kernels with water and drain well. Place the rice in a medium saucepan with a tight fitting lid, along with the water, coconut milk, salt and freshly ground black pepper. Bring the mixture to a boil and then cover, reduce the heat and let it cook gently for 20 minutes without lifting the lid. When the time is up, lift the lid, fluff with a fork and set aside.
6. Remove the chicken from the air fryer and serve warm with the coconut rice and fresh cilantro scattered around.

Lemon Sage Roast Chicken

Servings: 4

Cooking Time: 60 Minutes

Ingredients:

- 1 (4-pound) chicken
- 1 bunch sage, divided
- 1 lemon, zest and juice
- salt and freshly ground black pepper

Directions:

1. Preheat the air fryer to 350°F and pour a little water into the bottom of the air fryer drawer. (This will help prevent the grease that drips into the bottom drawer from burning and smoking.)
2. Run your fingers between the skin and flesh of the chicken breasts and thighs. Push a couple of sage leaves up underneath the skin of the chicken on each breast and each thigh.
3. Push some of the lemon zest up under the skin of the chicken next to the sage. Sprinkle some of the zest inside the chicken cavity, and reserve any leftover zest. Squeeze the lemon juice all over the chicken and in the cavity as well.
4. Season the chicken, inside and out, with the salt and freshly ground black pepper. Set a few sage leaves aside for the final garnish. Crumple up the remaining sage leaves and push them into the cavity of the chicken, along with one of the squeezed lemon halves.
5. Place the chicken breast side up into the air fryer basket and air-fry for 20 minutes at 350°F. Flip the chicken over so that it is breast side down and continue to air-fry for another 20 minutes. Return the chicken to breast side up and finish air-frying for 20 more minutes. The internal temperature of the chicken should register 165°F in the thickest part of the thigh when fully cooked. Remove the chicken from the air fryer and let it rest on a cutting board for at least 5 minutes.
6. Cut the rested chicken into pieces, sprinkle with the reserved lemon zest and garnish with the reserved sage leaves.

Teriyaki Chicken Legs

Servings: 2

Cooking Time: 20 Minutes

Ingredients:

- 4 tablespoons teriyaki sauce
- 1 tablespoon orange juice
- 1 teaspoon smoked paprika
- 4 chicken legs
- cooking spray

Directions:

1. Mix together the teriyaki sauce, orange juice, and smoked paprika. Brush on all sides of chicken legs.
2. Spray air fryer basket with nonstick cooking spray and place chicken in basket.
3. Cook at 360°F for 6minutes. Turn and baste with sauce. Cook for 6 moreminutes, turn and baste.

Cook for 8 minutes more, until juices run clear when chicken is pierced with a fork.

Tandoori Chicken Legs

Servings: 2

Cooking Time: 30 Minutes

Ingredients:

- 1 cup plain yogurt
- 2 cloves garlic, minced
- 1 tablespoon grated fresh ginger
- 2 teaspoons paprika
- 2 teaspoons ground coriander
- 1 teaspoon ground turmeric
- 1 teaspoon salt
- ¼ teaspoon ground cayenne pepper
- juice of 1 lime
- 2 bone-in, skin-on chicken legs
- fresh cilantro leaves

Directions:

1. Make the marinade by combining the yogurt, garlic, ginger, spices and lime juice. Make slashes into the chicken legs to help the marinade penetrate the meat. Pour the marinade over the chicken legs, cover and let the chicken marinate for at least an hour or overnight in the refrigerator.
2. Preheat the air fryer to 380°F.
3. Transfer the chicken legs from the marinade to the air fryer basket, reserving any extra marinade. Air-fry for 15 minutes. Flip the chicken over and pour the remaining marinade over the top. Air-fry for another 15 minutes, watching to make sure it doesn't brown too much. If it does start to get too brown, you can loosely tent the chicken with aluminum foil, tucking the ends of the foil under the chicken to stop it from blowing around.
4. Serve over rice with some fresh cilantro on top.

BEEF , PORK & LAMB RECIPES

Wasabi-coated Pork Loin Chops

Servings: 3

Cooking Time: 14 Minutes

Ingredients:

- 1½ cups Wasabi peas
- ¼ cup Plain panko bread crumbs
- 1 Large egg white(s)
- 2 tablespoons Water
- 3 5- to 6-ounce boneless center-cut pork loin chops (about ½ inch thick)

Directions:

1. Preheat the air fryer to 375°F .
2. Put the wasabi peas in a food processor. Cover and process until finely ground, about like panko bread crumbs. Add the bread crumbs and pulse a few times to blend.
3. Set up and fill two shallow soup plates or small pie plates on your counter: one for the egg white(s), whisked with the water until uniform; and one for the wasabi pea mixture.
4. Dip a pork chop in the egg white mixture, coating the chop on both sides as well as around the edge. Allow any excess egg white mixture to slip back into the rest, then set the chop in the wasabi pea mixture. Press gently and turn it several times to coat evenly on both sides and around the edge. Set aside, then dip and coat the remaining chop(s).
5. Set the chops in the basket with as much air space between them as possible. Air-fry, turning once at the 6-minute mark, for 12 minutes, or until the chops are crisp and browned and an instant-read meat thermometer inserted into the center of a chop registers 145°F. If the machine is at 360°F, you may need to add 2 minutes to the cooking time.
6. Use kitchen tongs to transfer the chops to a wire rack. Cool for a couple of minutes before serving.

Crispy Ham And Eggs

Servings: 3

Cooking Time: 9 Minutes

Ingredients:

- 2 cups Rice-puff cereal, such as Rice Krispies
- ¼ cup Maple syrup
- ½ pound ¼- to ½-inch-thick ham steak (gluten-free, if a concern)
- 1 tablespoon Unsalted butter
- 3 Large eggs
- ⅛ teaspoon Table salt
- ⅛ teaspoon Ground black pepper

Directions:

1. Preheat the air fryer to 400°F.
2. Pour the cereal into a food processor, cover, and process until finely ground. Pour the ground cereal into a shallow soup plate or a small pie plate.
3. Smear the maple syrup on both sides of the ham, then set the ham into the ground cereal. Turn a few times, pressing gently, until evenly coated.
4. Set the ham steak in the basket and air-fry undisturbed for 5 minutes, or until browned.
5. Meanwhile, melt the butter in a medium or large nonstick skillet set over medium heat. Crack the eggs into the skillet and cook until the whites are set and the yolks are hot, about 3 minutes (or 4 minutes for a more set yolk.) Season with the salt and pepper.
6. When the ham is ready, transfer it to a serving platter, then slip the eggs from the skillet on top of it. Divide into portions to serve.

Bacon Wrapped Filets Mignons

Servings: 4

Cooking Time: 18 Minutes

Ingredients:

- 4 slices bacon (not thick cut)
- 4 (8-ounce) filets mignons
- 1 tablespoon fresh thyme leaves
- salt and freshly ground black pepper

Directions:

1. Preheat the air fryer to 400°F.
2. Lay the bacon slices down on a cutting board and sprinkle the thyme leaves on the bacon slices. Remove any string tying the filets and place the steaks down on their sides on top of the bacon slices. Roll the bacon around the side of the filets and secure the bacon to the fillets with a toothpick or two.
3. Season the steaks generously with salt and freshly ground black pepper and transfer the steaks to the air fryer.
4. Air-fry for 18 minutes, turning the steaks over halfway through the cooking process. This should cook your steaks to about medium, depending on how thick they are. If you'd prefer your steaks medium-rare or medium-well, simply add or subtract two minutes from the cooking time. Remove the steaks from the air fryer and let them rest for 5 minutes before removing the toothpicks and serving. (Just enough time to quickly air-fry some vegetables to go with them!)

Apple Cornbread Stuffed Pork Loin With Apple Gravy

Servings: 4

Cooking Time: 61 Minutes

Ingredients:

- 4 strips of bacon, chopped
- 1 Granny Smith apple, peeled, cored and finely chopped
- 2 teaspoons fresh thyme leaves
- ¼ cup chopped fresh parsley
- 2 cups cubed cornbread
- ½ cup chicken stock
- salt and freshly ground black pepper
- 1 (2-pound) boneless pork loin
- kitchen twine
- Apple Gravy:
- 2 tablespoons butter
- 1 shallot, minced
- 1 Granny Smith apple, peeled, cored and finely chopped
- 3 sprigs fresh thyme
- 2 tablespoons flour
- 1 cup chicken stock
- ½ cup apple cider
- salt and freshly ground black pepper, to taste

Directions:

1. Preheat the air fryer to 400°F.
2. Add the bacon to the air fryer and air-fry for 6 minutes until crispy. While the bacon is cooking, combine the apple, fresh thyme, parsley and cornbread in a bowl and toss well. Moisten the mixture with the chicken stock and season to taste with salt and freshly ground black pepper. Add the cooked bacon to the mixture.
3. Butterfly the pork loin by holding it flat on the cutting board with one hand, while slicing into the pork loin parallel to the cutting board with the other. Slice into the longest side of the pork loin, but stop before you cut all the way through. You should then be able to open the pork loin up like a book, making it twice as wide as it was when you started. Season the inside of the pork with salt and freshly ground black pepper.
4. Spread the cornbread mixture onto the butterflied pork loin, leaving a one-inch border around the edge of the pork. Roll the pork loin up around the stuffing to enclose the stuffing, and tie the rolled pork in several places with kitchen twine or secure with toothpicks. Try to replace any stuffing that falls out of the roast as you roll it, by stuffing it into the ends of the rolled pork. Season the outside of the pork with salt and freshly ground black pepper.
5. Preheat the air fryer to 360°F.
6. Place the stuffed pork loin into the air fryer, seam side down. Air-fry the pork loin for 15 minutes at 360°F. Turn the pork loin over and air-fry for an additional 15 minutes. Turn the pork loin a quarter turn and air-fry for an additional 15 minutes. Turn the pork loin over again to expose the fourth side,

and air-fry for an additional 10 minutes. The pork loin should register 155°F on an instant read thermometer when it is finished.

7. While the pork is cooking, make the apple gravy. Preheat a saucepan over medium heat on the stovetop and melt the butter. Add the shallot, apple and thyme sprigs and sauté until the apple starts to soften and brown a little. Add the flour and stir for a minute or two. Whisk in the stock and apple cider vigorously to prevent the flour from forming lumps. Bring the mixture to a boil to thicken and season to taste with salt and pepper.

8. Transfer the pork loin to a resting plate and loosely tent with foil, letting the pork rest for at least 5 minutes before slicing and serving with the apple gravy poured over the top.

Sloppy Joes

Servings: 4 Cooking Time: 17 Minutes

Ingredients:

- oil for misting or cooking spray
- 1 pound very lean ground beef
- 1 teaspoon onion powder
- ⅓ cup ketchup
- ¼ cup water
- ½ teaspoon celery seed
- 1 tablespoon lemon juice
- 1½ teaspoons brown sugar
- 1¼ teaspoons low-sodium Worcestershire sauce
- ½ teaspoon salt (optional)
- ½ teaspoon vinegar
- ⅛ teaspoon dry mustard
- hamburger or slider buns

Directions:

1. Spray air fryer basket with nonstick cooking spray or olive oil.
2. Break raw ground beef into small chunks and pile into basket.
3. Cook at 390°F for 5minutes. Stir to break apart and cook 3minutes. Stir and cook 4 minutes longer or until meat is well done.
4. Remove meat from air fryer, drain, and use a knife and fork to crumble into small pieces.
5. Give your air fryer basket a quick rinse to remove any bits of meat.
6. Place all the remaining ingredients except the buns in a 6 x 6-inch baking pan and mix together.
7. Add meat and stir well.
8. Cook at 330°F for 5minutes. Stir and cook for 2minutes.
9. Scoop onto buns.

Pepperoni Pockets

Servings: 4

Cooking Time: 8 Minutes

Ingredients:

- 4 bread slices, 1-inch thick
- olive oil for misting
- 24 slices pepperoni (about 2 ounces)
- 1 ounce roasted red peppers, drained and patted dry
- 1 ounce Pepper Jack cheese cut into 4 slices
- pizza sauce (optional)

Directions:

1. Spray both sides of bread slices with olive oil.
2. Stand slices upright and cut a deep slit in the top to create a pocket—almost to the bottom crust but not all the way through.
3. Stuff each bread pocket with 6 slices of pepperoni, a large strip of roasted red pepper, and a slice of cheese.
4. Place bread pockets in air fryer basket, standing up. Cook at 360°F for 8 minutes, until filling is heated through and bread is lightly browned. Serve while hot as is or with pizza sauce for dipping.

Chicken-fried Steak

Servings: 2

Cooking Time: 12 Minutes

Ingredients:

- 1½ cups All-purpose flour
- 2 Large egg(s)
- 2 tablespoons Regular or low-fat sour cream
- 2 tablespoons Worcestershire sauce
- 2 ¼-pound thin beef cube steak(s)
- Vegetable oil spray

Directions:

1. Preheat the air fryer to 400°F.
2. Set up and fill two shallow soup plates or small pie plates on your counter: one for the flour; and one for the egg(s), whisked with the sour cream and Worcestershire sauce until uniform.
3. Dredge a piece of beef in the flour, coating it well on both sides and even along the edge. Shake off any excess; then dip the meat in the egg mixture, coating both sides while retaining the flour on the meat. Let any excess egg mixture slip back into the rest. Dredge the meat in the flour once again, coating all surfaces well. Gently shake off the excess coating and set the steak aside if you're coating another steak or two. Once done, coat the steak(s) on both sides with the vegetable oil spray.
4. Set the steak(s) in the basket. If there's more than one steak, make sure they do not overlap or even touch, although the smallest gap between them is enough to get them crunchy. Air-fry undisturbed for 6 minutes.
5. Use kitchen tongs to pick up one of the steaks. Coat it again on both sides with vegetable oil spray. Turn it upside down and set it back in the basket with that same regard for the space between them in larger batches. Repeat with any other steaks. Continue air-frying undisturbed for 6 minutes, or until golden brown and crunchy.
6. Use kitchen tongs to transfer the steak(s) to a wire rack. Cool for 5 minutes before serving.

Chicken Fried Steak

Servings: 4

Cooking Time: 15 Minutes

Ingredients:

- 2 eggs
- ½ cup buttermilk
- 1½ cups flour
- ¾ teaspoon salt
- ½ teaspoon pepper
- 1 pound beef cube steaks
- salt and pepper
- oil for misting or cooking spray

Directions:

1. Beat together eggs and buttermilk in a shallow dish.
2. In another shallow dish, stir together the flour, ½ teaspoon salt, and ¼ teaspoon pepper.
3. Season cube steaks with remaining salt and pepper to taste. Dip in flour, buttermilk egg wash, and then flour again.
4. Spray both sides of steaks with oil or cooking spray.
5. Cooking in 2 batches, place steaks in air fryer basket in single layer. Cook at 360°F for 10minutes. Spray tops of steaks with oil and cook 5minutes or until meat is well done.
6. Repeat to cook remaining steaks.

Pork & Beef Egg Rolls

Servings: 8

Cooking Time: 8 Minutes

Ingredients:

- ¼ pound very lean ground beef
- ¼ pound lean ground pork
- 1 tablespoon soy sauce
- 1 teaspoon olive oil
- ½ cup grated carrots
- 2 green onions, chopped
- 2 cups grated Napa cabbage
- ¼ cup chopped water chestnuts
- ¼ teaspoon salt
- ¼ teaspoon garlic powder
- ¼ teaspoon black pepper
- 1 egg
- 1 tablespoon water
- 8 egg roll wraps
- oil for misting or cooking spray

Directions:

1. In a large skillet, brown beef and pork with soy sauce. Remove cooked meat from skillet, drain, and set aside.
2. Pour off any excess grease from skillet. Add olive oil, carrots, and onions. Sauté until barely tender, about 1 minute.
3. Stir in cabbage, cover, and cook for 1 minute or just until cabbage slightly wilts. Remove from heat.
4. In a large bowl, combine the cooked meats and vegetables, water chestnuts, salt, garlic powder, and pepper. Stir well. If needed, add more salt to taste.
5. Beat together egg and water in a small bowl.
6. Fill egg roll wrappers, using about ¼ cup of filling for each wrap. Roll up and brush all over with egg wash to seal. Spray very lightly with olive oil or cooking spray.
7. Place 4 egg rolls in air fryer basket and cook at 390°F for 4minutes. Turn over and cook 4 more minutes, until golden brown and crispy.
8. Repeat to cook remaining egg rolls.

California Burritos

Servings: 4

Cooking Time: 17 Minutes

Ingredients:

- 1 pound sirloin steak, sliced thin
- 1 teaspoon dried oregano
- 1 teaspoon ground cumin
- ½ teaspoon garlic powder
- 16 tater tots
- ⅓ cup sour cream
- ½ lime, juiced
- 2 tablespoons hot sauce
- 1 large avocado, pitted
- 1 teaspoon salt, divided
- 4 large (8- to 10-inch) flour tortillas
- ½ cup shredded cheddar cheese or Monterey jack
- 2 tablespoons avocado oil

Directions:

1. Preheat the air fryer to 380°F.
2. Season the steak with oregano, cumin, and garlic powder. Place the steak on one side of the air fryer and the tater tots on the other side. (It's okay for them to touch, because the flavors will all come together in the burrito.) Cook for 8 minutes, toss, and cook an additional 4 to 6 minutes.
3. Meanwhile, in a small bowl, stir together the sour cream, lime juice, and hot sauce.
4. In another small bowl, mash together the avocado and season with ½ teaspoon of the salt, to taste.
5. To assemble the burrito, lay out the tortillas, equally divide the meat amongst the tortillas. Season the steak equally with the remaining ½ teaspoon salt. Then layer the mashed avocado and sour cream mixture on top. Top each tortilla with 4 tater tots and finish each with 2 tablespoons cheese. Roll up the sides and, while holding in the sides, roll up the burrito. Place the burritos in the air fryer basket and brush with avocado oil (working in batches as needed); cook for 3 minutes or until lightly golden on the outside.

Cinnamon-stick Kofta Skewers

Servings: 8

Cooking Time: 15 Minutes

Ingredients:

- 1 pound Lean ground beef
- ½ teaspoon Ground cumin
- ½ teaspoon Onion powder
- ½ teaspoon Ground dried turmeric
- ½ teaspoon Ground cinnamon
- ½ teaspoon Table salt
- Up to a ⅛ teaspoon Cayenne
- 8 3½- to 4-inch-long cinnamon sticks (see the headnote)
- Vegetable oil spray

Directions:

1. Preheat the air fryer to 375°F .
2. Gently mix the ground beef, cumin, onion powder, turmeric, cinnamon, salt, and cayenne in a bowl until the meat is evenly mixed with the spices. (Clean, dry hands work best!) Divide this mixture into 2-ounce portions, each about the size of a golf ball.
3. Wrap one portion of the meat mixture around a cinnamon stick, using about three-quarters of the length of the stick, covering one end but leaving a little "handle" of cinnamon stick protruding from the other end. Set aside and continue making more kofta skewers.
4. Generously coat the formed kofta skewers on all sides with vegetable oil spray. Set them in the basket with as much air space between them as possible. Air-fry undisturbed for 13 minutes, or until browned and cooked through. If the machine is at 360°F, you may need to add 2 minutes to the cooking time.
5. Use a nonstick-safe spatula, and perhaps kitchen tongs for balance, to gently transfer the kofta skewers to a wire rack. Cool for at least 5 minutes or up to 20 minutes before serving.

Honey Mesquite Pork Chops

Servings: 2

Cooking Time: 10 Minutes

Ingredients:

- 2 tablespoons mesquite seasoning
- ¼ cup honey
- 1 tablespoon olive oil
- 1 tablespoon water
- freshly ground black pepper
- 2 bone-in center cut pork chops (about 1 pound)

Directions:

1. Whisk the mesquite seasoning, honey, olive oil, water and freshly ground black pepper together in a shallow glass dish. Pierce the chops all over and on both sides with a fork or meat tenderizer. Add the pork chops to the marinade and massage the marinade into the chops. Cover and marinate for 30 minutes.
2. Preheat the air fryer to 330°F.
3. Transfer the pork chops to the air fryer basket and pour half of the marinade over the chops, reserving the remaining marinade. Air-fry the pork chops for 6 minutes. Flip the pork chops over and pour the remaining marinade on top. Air-fry for an additional 3 minutes at 330°F. Then, increase the air fryer temperature to 400°F and air-fry the pork chops for an additional minute.
4. Transfer the pork chops to a serving plate, and let them rest for 5 minutes before serving. If you'd like a sauce for these chops, pour the cooked marinade from the bottom of the air fryer over the top.

APPETIZERS AND SNACKS

Eggs In Avocado Halves

Servings: 3

Cooking Time: 23 Minutes

Ingredients:

- 3 Hass avocados, halved and pitted but not peeled
- 6 Medium eggs
- Vegetable oil spray
- 3 tablespoons Heavy or light cream (not fat-free cream)
- To taste Table salt
- To taste Ground black pepper

Directions:

1. Preheat the air fryer to 350°F .
2. Slice a small amount off the (skin) side of each avocado half so it can sit stable, without rocking. Lightly coat the skin of the avocado half (the side that will now sit stable) with vegetable oil spray.
3. Arrange the avocado halves open side up on a cutting board, then crack an egg into the indentation in each where the pit had been. If any white overflows the avocado half, wipe that bit of white off the cut edge of the avocado before proceeding.
4. Remove the basket (or its attachment) from the machine and set the filled avocado halves in it in one layer. Return it to the machine without pushing it in. Drizzle each avocado half with about 1½ teaspoons cream, a little salt, and a little ground black pepper.
5. Air-fry undisturbed for 10 minutes for a soft-set yolk, or air-fry for 13 minutes for more-set eggs.
6. Use a nonstick-safe spatula and a flatware fork for balance to transfer the avocado halves to serving plates. Cool a minute or two before serving.

Fried Pickles

Servings: 2

Cooking Time: 15 Minutes

Ingredients:

- 1 egg
- 1 tablespoon milk
- ¼ teaspoon hot sauce
- 2 cups sliced dill pickles, well drained
- ¾ cup breadcrumbs
- oil for misting or cooking spray

Directions:

1. Preheat air fryer to 390°F.
2. Beat together egg, milk, and hot sauce in a bowl large enough to hold all the pickles.
3. Add pickles to the egg wash and stir well to coat.
4. Place breadcrumbs in a large plastic bag or container with lid.
5. Drain egg wash from pickles and place them in bag with breadcrumbs. Shake to coat.
6. Pile pickles into air fryer basket and spray with oil.
7. Cook for 5minutes. Shake basket and spray with oil.
8. Cook 5 more minutes. Shake and spray again. Separate any pickles that have stuck together and mist any spots you've missed.
9. Cook for 5minutes longer or until dark golden brown and crispy.

Classic Potato Chips

Servings: 4

Cooking Time: 8 Minutes

Ingredients:

- 2 medium russet potatoes, washed
- 2 cups filtered water
- 1 tablespoon avocado oil
- ½ teaspoon salt

Directions:

1. Using a mandolin, slice the potatoes into ⅛-inch-thick pieces.
2. Pour the water into a large bowl. Place the potatoes in the bowl and soak for at least 30 minutes.
3. Preheat the air fryer to 350°F.
4. Drain the water and pat the potatoes dry with a paper towel or kitchen cloth. Toss with avocado oil and salt. Liberally spray the air fryer basket with olive oil mist.
5. Set the potatoes inside the air fryer basket, separating them so they're not on top of each other. Cook for 5 minutes, shake the basket, and cook another 5 minutes, or until browned.
6. Remove and let cool a few minutes prior to serving. Repeat until all the chips are cooked.

Spanakopita Spinach, Feta And Pine Nut Phyllo Bites

Servings: 8

Cooking Time: 10 Minutes

Ingredients:

- ½ (10-ounce) package frozen spinach, thawed and squeezed dry (about 1 cup)
- ¾ cup crumbled feta cheese
- ¼ cup grated Parmesan cheese
- ¼ cup pine nuts, toasted
- ⅛ teaspoon ground nutmeg
- 1 egg, lightly beaten
- ½ teaspoon salt
- freshly ground black pepper
- 6 sheets phyllo dough
- ½ cup butter, melted

Directions:

1. Combine the spinach, cheeses, pine nuts, nutmeg and egg in a bowl. Season with salt and freshly ground black pepper.
2. While building the phyllo triangles, always keep the dough sheets you are not working with covered with plastic wrap and a damp clean kitchen towel. Remove one sheet of the phyllo and place it on a flat surface. Brush the phyllo sheet with melted butter and then layer another sheet of phyllo on top. Brush the second sheet of phyllo with butter. Cut the layered phyllo sheets into 6 strips, about 2½- to 3-inches wide.
3. Place a heaping tablespoon of the spinach filling at the end of each strip of dough. Fold the bottom right corner of the strip over the filling towards the left edge of the strip to make a triangle. Continue to fold the phyllo dough around the spinach as you would fold a flag, making triangle after triangle. Brush the outside of the phyllo triangle with more melted butter and set it aside until you've finished the 6 strips of dough, making 6 triangles.
4. Preheat the air fryer to 350°F.
5. Transfer the first six phyllo triangles to the air fryer basket and air-fry for 5 minutes. Turn the triangles over and air-fry for another 5 minutes.
6. While the first batch of triangles is air-frying, build another set of triangles and air-fry in the same manner. You should do three batches total. These can be warmed in the air fryer for a minute or two just before serving if you like.

Country Wings

Servings: 4

Cooking Time: 19 Minutes

Ingredients:

- 2 pounds chicken wings
- Marinade
- 1 cup buttermilk
- ½ teaspoon black pepper
- ½ teaspoon salt
- Coating
- 1 cup flour
- 1 cup panko breadcrumbs
- 2 teaspoons salt
- 2 tablespoons poultry seasoning
- oil for misting or cooking spray

Directions:

1. Cut the tips off the wings. Discard or freeze for stock. Cut remaining wing sections apart at the joint to make 2 pieces per wing. Place wings in a large bowl or plastic bag.
2. Mix together all marinade ingredients and pour over wings. Refrigerate for at least 1 hour but for no more than 8 hours.
3. Preheat air fryer to 360°F.
4. Mix all coating ingredients together in a shallow dish or on wax paper.
5. Remove wings from marinade, shaking off excess, and roll in coating mixture.
6. Spray both sides of each wing with oil or cooking spray.
7. Place wings in air fryer basket in single layer, close but not too crowded. Cook for 19minutes or until chicken is done and juices run clear.
8. Repeat step 7 to cook remaining wings.

Sausage And Cheese Rolls

Servings: 3

Cooking Time: 18 Minutes

Ingredients:

- 3 3- to 3½-ounce sweet or hot Italian sausage links
- 2 1-ounce string cheese stick(s), unwrapped and cut in half lengthwise
- Three quarters from one thawed sheet (cut the sheet into four quarters; wrap and refreeze one of them) A 17.25-ounce box frozen puff pastry

Directions:

1. Preheat the air fryer to 400°F.
2. When the machine is at temperature, set the sausage links in the basket and air-fry undisturbed for 12 minutes, or until cooked through.
3. Use kitchen tongs to transfer the links to a wire rack. Cool for 15 minutes. (If necessary, pour out any rendered fat that has collected below the basket in the machine.)
4. Cut the sausage links in half lengthwise. Sandwich half a string cheese stick between two sausage halves, trimming the ends so the cheese doesn't stick out beyond the meat.
5. Roll each piece of puff pastry into a 6 x 6-inch square on a clean, dry work surface. Set the sausage-cheese sandwich at one edge and roll it up in the dough. The ends will be open like a pig-in-a-blanket. Repeat with the remaining puff pastry, sausage, and cheese.
6. Set the rolls seam side down in the basket. Air-fry undisturbed for 6 minutes, or until puffed and golden brown.
7. Use a nonstick-safe spatula, and perhaps a flatware fork for balance, to transfer the rolls to a wire rack. Cool for at least 5 minutes before serving.

Fried Goat Cheese

Servings: 3

Cooking Time: 4 Minutes

Ingredients:

- 7 ounces 1- to 1½-inch-diameter goat cheese log
- 2 Large egg(s)
- 1¾ cups Plain dried bread crumbs (gluten-free, if a concern)
- Vegetable oil spray

Directions:

1. Slice the goat cheese log into ½-inch-thick rounds. Set these flat on a small cutting board, a small baking sheet, or a large plate. Freeze uncovered for 30 minutes.
2. Preheat the air fryer to 400°F.
3. Set up and fill two shallow soup plates or small pie plates on your counter: one in which you whisk the egg(s) until uniform and the other for the bread crumbs.
4. Take the goat cheese rounds out of the freezer. With clean, dry hands, dip one round in the egg(s) to coat it on all sides. Let the excess egg slip back into the rest, then dredge the round in the bread crumbs, turning it to coat all sides, even the edges. Repeat this process—egg, then bread crumbs—for a second coating. Coat both sides of the round and its edges with vegetable oil spray, then set it aside. Continue double-dipping, double-dredging, and spraying the remaining rounds.
5. Place the rounds in one layer in the basket. Air-fry undisturbed for 4 minutes, or until lightly browned and crunchy. Do not overcook. Some of the goat cheese may break through the crust. A few little breaks are fine but stop the cooking before the coating reaches structural failure.
6. Remove the basket from the machine and set aside for 3 minutes. Use a nonstick-safe spatula, and maybe a flatware fork for balance, to transfer the rounds to a wire rack. Cool for 5 minutes more before serving.

Smoked Salmon Puffs

Servings: 2

Cooking Time: 8 Minutes

Ingredients:

- Two quarters of one thawed sheet (that is, a half of the sheet; wrap and refreeze the remainder) A 17.25-ounce box frozen puff pastry
- 4 ½-ounce smoked salmon slices
- 2 tablespoons Softened regular or low-fat cream cheese (not fat-free)
- Up to 2 teaspoons Drained and rinsed capers, minced
- Up to 2 teaspoons Minced red onion
- 1 Large egg white
- 1 tablespoon Water

Directions:

1. Preheat the air fryer to 400°F.
2. For a small air fryer, roll the piece of puff pastry into a 6 x 6-inch square on a clean, dry work surface.
3. For a medium or larger air fryer, roll each piece of puff pastry into a 6 x 6-inch square.
4. Set 2 salmon slices on the diagonal, corner to corner, on each rolled-out sheet. Smear the salmon with cream cheese, then sprinkle with capers and red onion. Fold the sheet closed by picking up one corner that does not have an edge of salmon near it and folding the dough across the salmon to its opposite corner. Seal the edges closed by pressing the tines of a flatware fork into them.
5. Whisk the egg white and water in a small bowl until uniform. Brush this mixture over the top(s) of the packet(s).
6. Set the packet(s) in the basket (if you're working with more than one, they cannot touch). Air-fry undisturbed for 8 minutes, or until golden brown and flaky.
7. Use a nonstick-safe spatula to transfer the packet(s) to a wire rack. Cool for 5 minutes before serving.

Mozzarella En Carrozza With Puttanesca Sauce

Servings: 6

Cooking Time: 8 Minutes

Ingredients:

- Puttanesca Sauce
- 2 teaspoons olive oil
- 1 anchovy, chopped (optional)
- 2 cloves garlic, minced
- 1 (14-ounce) can petite diced tomatoes
- ½ cup chicken stock or water
- ⅓ cup Kalamata olives, chopped
- 2 tablespoons capers
- ½ teaspoon dried oregano
- ¼ teaspoon crushed red pepper flakes
- salt and freshly ground black pepper
- 1 tablespoon fresh parsley, chopped
- 8 slices of thinly sliced white bread (Pepperidge Farm®)
- 8 ounces mozzarella cheese, cut into ¼-inch slices
- ½ cup all-purpose flour
- 3 eggs, beaten
- 1½ cups seasoned panko breadcrumbs
- ½ teaspoon garlic powder
- ½ teaspoon salt
- freshly ground black pepper
- olive oil, in a spray bottle

Directions:

1. Start by making the puttanesca sauce. Heat the olive oil in a medium saucepan on the stovetop. Add the anchovies (if using, and I really think you should!) and garlic and sauté for 3 minutes, or until the anchovies have "melted" into the oil. Add the tomatoes, chicken stock, olives, capers, oregano and crushed red pepper flakes and simmer the sauce for 20 minutes. Season with salt and freshly ground black pepper and stir in the fresh parsley.
2. Cut the crusts off the slices of bread. Place four slices of the bread on a cutting board. Divide the cheese between the four slices of bread. Top the cheese with the remaining four slices of bread to make little sandwiches and cut each sandwich into 4 triangles.
3. Set up a dredging station using three shallow dishes. Place the flour in the first shallow dish, the eggs in the second dish and in the third dish, combine the panko breadcrumbs, garlic powder, salt and black pepper. Dredge each little triangle in the flour first (you might think this is redundant, but it helps to get the coating to adhere to the edges of the sandwiches) and then dip them into the egg, making sure both the sides and the edges are coated. Let the excess egg drip off and then press the triangles into the breadcrumb mixture, pressing the crumbs on with your hands so they adhere. Place the coated triangles in the freezer for 2 hours, until the cheese is frozen.
4. Preheat the air fryer to 390°F. Spray all sides of the mozzarella triangles with oil and transfer a single layer of triangles to the air fryer basket. Air-fry in batches at 390°F for 5 minutes. Turn the triangles over and air-fry for an additional 3 minutes.
5. Serve mozzarella triangles immediately with the warm puttanesca sauce.

Potato Chips With Sour Cream And Onion Dip

Servings: 2

Cooking Time: 20 Minutes

Ingredients:

- 2 large potatoes (Yukon Gold or russet)
- vegetable or olive oil in a spray bottle
- sea salt and freshly ground black pepper
- Sour Cream and Onion Dip:
- ½ cup sour cream
- 1 tablespoon olive oil
- 2 scallions, white part only minced
- ¼ teaspoon salt
- freshly ground black pepper
- a squeeze of lemon juice (about ¼ teaspoon)

Directions:

1. Wash the potatoes well, but leave the skins on. Slice them into ⅛-inch thin slices, using a mandolin or food processor. Rinse the potatoes under cold water until the water runs clear and then let them soak in a bowl of cold water for at least 10 minutes. Drain and dry the potato slices really well in a single layer on a clean kitchen towel.
2. Preheat the air fryer to 300°F. Spray the potato chips with the oil so that both sides are evenly coated, or rub the slices between your hands with some oil if you don't have a spray bottle.
3. Air-fry in two batches at 300°F for 20 minutes, shaking the basket a few times during the cooking process so the chips crisp and brown more evenly. Season the finished chips with sea salt and freshly ground black pepper while they are still hot.
4. While the chips are air-frying, make the sour cream and onion dip by mixing together the sour cream, olive oil, scallions, salt, pepper and lemon juice. Serve the chips warm or at room temperature along with the dip.

Cuban Sliders

Servings: 8

Cooking Time: 8 Minutes

Ingredients:

- 8 slices ciabatta bread, ¼-inch thick
- cooking spray
- 1 tablespoon brown mustard
- 6-8 ounces thin sliced leftover roast pork
- 4 ounces thin deli turkey
- ⅓ cup bread and butter pickle slices
- 2–3 ounces Pepper Jack cheese slices

Directions:

1. Spray one side of each slice of bread with butter or olive oil cooking spray.
2. Spread brown mustard on other side of each slice.
3. Layer pork roast, turkey, pickles, and cheese on 4 of the slices. Top with remaining slices.
4. Cook at 390°F for approximately 8minutes. The sandwiches should be golden brown.
5. Cut each slider in half to make 8 portions.

Zucchini Fritters

Servings: 8

Cooking Time: 10 Minutes

Ingredients:

- 2 cups grated zucchini
- ½ teaspoon sea salt
- 1 egg
- ½ teaspoon garlic powder
- ¼ teaspoon onion powder
- ¼ cup grated Parmesan cheese
- ½ cup all-purpose flour
- ¼ teaspoon baking powder
- ½ cup Greek yogurt or sour cream
- ½ lime, juiced
- ¼ cup chopped cilantro
- ¼ teaspoon ground cumin
- ¼ teaspoon salt

Directions:

1. Preheat the air fryer to 360°F.
2. In a large colander, place a kitchen towel. Inside the towel, place the grated zucchini and sprinkle the sea salt over the top. Let the zucchini sit for 5 minutes; then, using the towel, squeeze dry the zucchini.
3. In a medium bowl, mix together the egg, garlic powder, onion powder, Parmesan cheese, flour, and baking powder. Add in the grated zucchini, and stir until completely combined.
4. Pierce a piece of parchment paper with a fork 4 to 6 times. Place the parchment paper into the air fryer basket. Using a tablespoon, place 6 to 8 heaping tablespoons of fritter batter onto the parchment paper. Spray the fritters with cooking spray and cook for 5 minutes, turn the fritters over, and cook another 5 minutes.
5. Meanwhile, while the fritters are cooking, make the sauce. In a small bowl, whisk together the Greek yogurt or sour cream, lime juice, cilantro, cumin, and salt.
6. Repeat Steps 2–4 with the remaining batter.

BREAD AND BREAKFAST

Quesadillas

Servings: 4

Cooking Time: 12 Minutes

Ingredients:

- 4 eggs
- 2 tablespoons skim milk
- salt and pepper
- oil for misting or cooking spray
- 4 flour tortillas
- 4 tablespoons salsa
- 2 ounces Cheddar cheese, grated
- ½ small avocado, peeled and thinly sliced

Directions:

1. Preheat air fryer to 270°F.
2. Beat together eggs, milk, salt, and pepper.
3. Spray a 6 x 6-inch air fryer baking pan lightly with cooking spray and add egg mixture.
4. Cook 9minutes, stirring every 1 to 2minutes, until eggs are scrambled to your liking. Remove and set aside.
5. Spray one side of each tortilla with oil or cooking spray. Flip over.
6. Divide eggs, salsa, cheese, and avocado among the tortillas, covering only half of each tortilla.
7. Fold each tortilla in half and press down lightly.
8. Place 2 tortillas in air fryer basket and cook at 390°F for 3minutes or until cheese melts and outside feels slightly crispy. Repeat with remaining two tortillas.
9. Cut each cooked tortilla into halves or thirds.

Parmesan Garlic Naan

Servings: 6

Cooking Time: 4 Minutes

Ingredients:

- 1 cup bread flour
- 1 teaspoon baking powder
- ⅛ teaspoon salt
- 1 teaspoon garlic powder
- 2 tablespoon shredded parmesan cheese
- 1 cup plain 2% fat Greek yogurt
- 1 tablespoon extra-virgin olive oil

Directions:

1. Preheat the air fryer to 400°F.
2. In a medium bowl, mix the flour, baking powder, salt, garlic powder, and cheese. Mix the yogurt into the flour, using your hands to combine if necessary.
3. On a flat surface covered with flour, divide the dough into 6 equal balls and roll each out into a 4-inch-diameter circle.
4. Lightly brush both sides of each naan with olive oil and place one naan at a time into the basket. Cook for 3 to 4 minutes (or until the bread begins to rise and brown on the outside). Remove and repeat for the remaining breads.
5. Serve warm.

Western Omelet

Servings: 2

Cooking Time: 22 Minutes

Ingredients:

- ¼ cup chopped onion
- ¼ cup chopped bell pepper, green or red
- ¼ cup diced ham
- 1 teaspoon butter
- 4 large eggs
- 2 tablespoons milk
- ⅛ teaspoon salt
- ¾ cup grated sharp Cheddar cheese

Directions:

1. Place onion, bell pepper, ham, and butter in air fryer baking pan. Cook at 390°F for 1 minute and stir. Continue cooking 5minutes, until vegetables are tender.
2. Beat together eggs, milk, and salt. Pour over vegetables and ham in baking pan. Cook at 360°F for 15minutes or until eggs set and top has browned slightly.
3. Sprinkle grated cheese on top of omelet. Cook 1 minute or just long enough to melt the cheese.

Green Onion Pancakes

Servings: 4

Cooking Time: 8 Minutes

Ingredients:

- 2 cup all-purpose flour
- ½ teaspoon salt
- ¾ cup hot water
- 1 tablespoon vegetable oil
- 1 tablespoon butter, melted
- 2 cups finely chopped green onions
- 1 tablespoon black sesame seeds, for garnish

Directions:

1. In a large bowl, whisk together the flour and salt. Make a well in the center and pour in the hot water. Quickly stir the flour mixture together until a dough forms. Knead the dough for 5 minutes; then cover with a warm, wet towel and set aside for 30 minutes to rest.
2. In a small bowl, mix together the vegetable oil and melted butter.
3. On a floured surface, place the dough and cut it into 8 pieces. Working with 1 piece of dough at a time, use a rolling pin to roll out the dough until it's ¼ inch thick; then brush the surface with the oil and butter mixture and sprinkle with green onions. Next, fold the dough in half and then in half again. Roll out the dough again until it's ¼ inch thick and brush with the oil and butter mixture and green onions. Fold the dough in half and then in half again and roll out one last time until it's ¼ inch thick. Repeat this technique with all 8 pieces.
4. Meanwhile, preheat the air fryer to 400°F.
5. Place 1 or 2 pancakes into the air fryer basket (or as many as will fit in your fryer), and cook for 2 minutes or until crispy and golden brown. Repeat until all the pancakes are cooked. Top with black sesame seeds for garnish, if desired.

Tuscan Toast

Servings: 4

Cooking Time: 5 Minutes

Ingredients:

- ¼ cup butter
- ½ teaspoon lemon juice
- ½ clove garlic
- ½ teaspoon dried parsley flakes
- 4 slices Italian bread, 1-inch thick

Directions:

1. Place butter, lemon juice, garlic, and parsley in a food processor. Process about 1 minute, or until garlic is pulverized and ingredients are well blended.
2. Spread garlic butter on both sides of bread slices.
3. Place bread slices upright in air fryer basket. (They can lie flat but cook better standing on end.)
4. Cook at 390°F for 5minutes or until toasty brown.

Farmers Market Quiche

Servings: 4

Cooking Time: 35 Minutes

Ingredients:

- 4 button mushrooms
- ¼ medium red bell pepper
- 1 teaspoon extra-virgin olive oil
- One 9-inch pie crust, at room temperature
- ¼ cup grated carrot
- ¼ cup chopped, fresh baby spinach leaves
- 3 eggs, whisked
- ¼ cup half-and-half
- ½ teaspoon thyme
- ½ teaspoon sea salt
- 2 ounces crumbled goat cheese or feta

Directions:

1. In a medium bowl, toss the mushrooms and bell pepper with extra-virgin olive oil; place into the air fryer basket. Set the temperature to 400°F for 8 minutes, stirring after 4 minutes. Remove from the air fryer, and roughly chop the mushrooms and bell peppers. Wipe the air fryer clean.
2. Prep a 7-inch oven-safe baking dish by spraying the bottom of the pan with cooking spray.
3. Place the pie crust into the baking dish; fold over and crimp the edges or use a fork to press to give the edges some shape.
4. In a medium bowl, mix together the mushrooms, bell peppers, carrots, spinach, and eggs. Stir in the half-and-half, thyme, and salt.
5. Pour the quiche mixture into the base of the pie shell. Top with crumbled cheese.
6. Place the quiche into the air fryer basket. Set the temperature to 325°F for 30 minutes.
7. When complete, turn the quiche halfway and cook an additional 5 minutes. Allow the quiche to rest 20 minutes prior to slicing and serving.

Broccoli Cornbread

Servings: 6

Cooking Time: 18 Minutes

Ingredients:

- 1 cup frozen chopped broccoli, thawed and drained
- ¼ cup cottage cheese
- 1 egg, beaten
- 2 tablespoons minced onion
- 2 tablespoons melted butter
- ½ cup flour
- ½ cup yellow cornmeal
- 1 teaspoon baking powder
- ½ teaspoon salt
- ¼ cup milk, plus 2 tablespoons
- cooking spray

Directions:

1. Place thawed broccoli in colander and press with a spoon to squeeze out excess moisture.
2. Stir together all ingredients in a large bowl.
3. Spray 6 x 6-inch baking pan with cooking spray.
4. Spread batter in pan and cook at 330°F for 18 minutes or until cornbread is lightly browned and loaf starts to pull away from sides of pan.

Coffee Cake

Servings: 8

Cooking Time: 35 Minutes

Ingredients:

- 4 tablespoons butter, melted and divided
- ⅓ cup cane sugar
- ¼ cup brown sugar
- 1 large egg
- 1 cup plus 6 teaspoons milk, divided
- 1 teaspoon vanilla extract
- 2 cups all-purpose flour
- 1½ teaspoons baking powder
- ¼ teaspoon salt
- 2 teaspoons ground cinnamon
- ⅓ cup chopped pecans
- ⅓ cup powdered sugar

Directions:

1. Preheat the air fryer to 325°F.
2. Using a hand mixer or stand mixer, in a medium bowl, cream together the butter, cane sugar, brown sugar, the egg, 1 cup of the milk, and the vanilla. Set aside.
3. In a small bowl, mix together the flour, baking powder, salt, and cinnamon. Slowly combine the dry ingredients into the wet. Fold in the pecans.
4. Liberally spray a 7-inch springform pan with cooking spray. Pour the batter into the pan and place in the air fryer basket.
5. Bake for 30 to 35 minutes. While the cake is baking, in a small bowl, add the powdered sugar and whisk together with the remaining 6 teaspoons of milk. Set aside.
6. When the cake is done baking, remove the pan from the basket and let cool on a wire rack. After 10 minutes, remove and invert the cake from pan. Drizzle with the powdered sugar glaze and serve.

Mini Pita Breads

Servings: 8

Cooking Time: 6 Minutes

Ingredients:

- 2 teaspoons active dry yeast
- 1 tablespoon sugar
- 1¼ to 1½ cups warm water (90° - 110°F)
- 3¼ cups all-purpose flour
- 2 teaspoons salt
- 1 tablespoon olive oil, plus more for brushing
- kosher salt (optional)

Directions:

1. Dissolve the yeast, sugar and water in the bowl of a stand mixer. Let the mixture sit for 5 minutes to make sure the yeast is active – it should foam a little. (If there's no foaming, discard and start again with new yeast.) Combine the flour and salt in a bowl, and add it to the water, along with the olive oil. Mix with the dough hook until combined. Add a little more flour if needed to get the dough to pull away from the sides of the mixing bowl, or add a little more water if the dough seems too dry.
2. Knead the dough until it is smooth and elastic (about 8 minutes in the mixer or 15 minutes by hand). Transfer the dough to a lightly oiled bowl, cover and let it rise in a warm place until doubled in bulk. Divide the dough into 8 portions and roll each portion into a circle about 4-inches in diameter. Don't roll the balls too thin, or you won't get the pocket inside the pita.
3. Preheat the air fryer to 400°F.
4. Brush both sides of the dough with olive oil, and sprinkle with kosher salt if desired. Air-fry one at a time at 400°F for 6 minutes, flipping it over when there are two minutes left in the cooking time.

Garlic Bread Knots

Servings: 8

Cooking Time: 5 Minutes

Ingredients:

- ¼ cup melted butter
- 2 teaspoons garlic powder
- 1 teaspoon dried parsley
- 1 (11-ounce) tube of refrigerated French bread dough

Directions:

1. Mix the melted butter, garlic powder and dried parsley in a small bowl and set it aside.
2. To make smaller knots, cut the long tube of bread dough into 16 slices. If you want to make bigger knots, slice the dough into 8 slices. Shape each slice into a long rope about 6 inches long by rolling it on a flat surface with the palm of your hands. Tie each rope into a knot and place them on a plate.
3. Preheat the air fryer to 350°F.
4. Transfer half of the bread knots into the air fryer basket, leaving space in between each knot. Brush each knot with the butter mixture using a pastry brush.
5. Air-fry for 5 minutes. Remove the baked knots and brush a little more of the garlic butter mixture on each. Repeat with the remaining bread knots and serve warm.

Walnut Pancake

Servings: 4

Cooking Time: 20 Minutes

Ingredients:

- 3 tablespoons butter, divided into thirds
- 1 cup flour
- 1½ teaspoons baking powder
- ¼ teaspoon salt
- 2 tablespoons sugar
- ¾ cup milk
- 1 egg, beaten
- 1 teaspoon pure vanilla extract
- ½ cup walnuts, roughly chopped
- maple syrup or fresh sliced fruit, for serving

Directions:

1. Place 1 tablespoon of the butter in air fryer baking pan. Cook at 330°F for 3minutes to melt.
2. In a small dish or pan, melt the remaining 2 tablespoons of butter either in the microwave or on the stove.
3. In a medium bowl, stir together the flour, baking powder, salt, and sugar. Add milk, beaten egg, the 2 tablespoons of melted butter, and vanilla. Stir until combined but do not beat. Batter may be slightly lumpy.
4. Pour batter over the melted butter in air fryer baking pan. Sprinkle nuts evenly over top.
5. Cook for 20minutes or until toothpick inserted in center comes out clean. Turn air fryer off, close the machine, and let pancake rest for 2minutes.
6. Remove pancake from pan, slice, and serve with syrup or fresh fruit.

Hush Puffins

Servings: 20

Cooking Time: 8 Minutes

Ingredients:

- 1 cup buttermilk
- ¼ cup butter, melted
- 2 eggs
- 1½ cups all-purpose flour
- 1½ cups cornmeal
- ⅓ cup sugar
- 1 teaspoon baking soda
- 1 teaspoon salt
- 4 scallions, minced
- vegetable oil

Directions:

1. Combine the buttermilk, butter and eggs in a large mixing bowl. In a second bowl combine the flour, cornmeal, sugar, baking soda and salt. Add the dry ingredients to the wet ingredients, stirring just to combine. Stir in the minced scallions and refrigerate the batter for 30 minutes.
2. Shape the batter into 2-inch balls. Brush or spray the balls with oil.
3. Preheat the air fryer to 360°F.
4. Air-fry the hush puffins in two batches at 360°F for 8 minutes, turning them over after 6 minutes of the cooking process.
5. Serve warm with butter.

VEGETARIANS RECIPES

Basic Fried Tofu

Servings: 4

Cooking Time: 17 Minutes

Ingredients:

- 14 ounces extra-firm tofu, drained and pressed
- 1 tablespoon sesame oil
- 2 tablespoons low-sodium soy sauce
- ¼ cup rice vinegar
- 1 tablespoon fresh grated ginger
- 1 clove garlic, minced
- 3 tablespoons cornstarch
- ¼ teaspoon black pepper
- ⅛ teaspoon salt

Directions:

1. Cut the tofu into 16 cubes. Set aside in a glass container with a lid.
2. In a medium bowl, mix the sesame oil, soy sauce, rice vinegar, ginger, and garlic. Pour over the tofu and secure the lid. Place in the refrigerator to marinate for an hour.
3. Preheat the air fryer to 350°F.
4. In a small bowl, mix the cornstarch, black pepper, and salt.
5. Transfer the tofu to a large bowl and discard the leftover marinade. Pour the cornstarch mixture over the tofu and toss until all the pieces are coated.
6. Liberally spray the air fryer basket with olive oil mist and set the tofu pieces inside. Allow space between the tofu so it can cook evenly. Cook in batches if necessary.
7. Cook 15 to 17 minutes, shaking the basket every 5 minutes to allow the tofu to cook evenly on all sides. When it's done cooking, the tofu will be crisped and browned on all sides.
8. Remove the tofu from the air fryer basket and serve warm.

Falafels

Servings: 12

Cooking Time: 10 Minutes

Ingredients:

- 1 pouch falafel mix
- 2–3 tablespoons plain breadcrumbs
- oil for misting or cooking spray

Directions:

1. Prepare falafel mix according to package directions.
2. Preheat air fryer to 390°F.
3. Place breadcrumbs in shallow dish or on wax paper.
4. Shape falafel mixture into 12 balls and flatten slightly. Roll in breadcrumbs to coat all sides and mist with oil or cooking spray.
5. Place falafels in air fryer basket in single layer and cook for 5minutes. Shake basket, and continue cooking for 5minutes, until they brown and are crispy.

Roasted Vegetable Thai Green Curry

Servings: 4

Cooking Time: 16 Minutes

Ingredients:

- 1 (13-ounce) can coconut milk
- 3 tablespoons green curry paste
- 1 tablespoon soy sauce*
- 1 tablespoon rice wine vinegar
- 1 teaspoon sugar
- 1 teaspoon minced fresh ginger
- ½ onion, chopped
- 3 carrots, sliced
- 1 red bell pepper, chopped
- olive oil
- 10 stalks of asparagus, cut into 2-inch pieces
- 3 cups broccoli florets
- basmati rice for serving
- fresh cilantro
- crushed red pepper flakes (optional)

Directions:

1. Combine the coconut milk, green curry paste, soy sauce, rice wine vinegar, sugar and ginger in a medium saucepan and bring to a boil on the stovetop. Reduce the heat and simmer for 20 minutes while you cook the vegetables. Set aside.
2. Preheat the air fryer to 400°F.
3. Toss the onion, carrots, and red pepper together with a little olive oil and transfer the vegetables to the air fryer basket. Air-fry at 400°F for 10 minutes, shaking the basket a few times during the cooking process. Add the asparagus and broccoli florets and air-fry for an additional 6 minutes, again shaking the basket for even cooking.
4. When the vegetables are cooked to your liking, toss them with the green curry sauce and serve in bowls over basmati rice. Garnish with fresh chopped cilantro and crushed red pepper flakes.

Mushroom And Fried Onion Quesadilla

Servings: 2

Cooking Time: 33 Minutes

Ingredients:

- 1 onion, sliced
- 2 tablespoons butter, melted
- 10 ounces button mushrooms, sliced
- 2 tablespoons Worcestershire sauce
- salt and freshly ground black pepper
- 4 (8-inch) flour tortillas
- 2 cups grated Fontina cheese
- vegetable or olive oil

Directions:

1. Preheat the air fryer to 400°F.
2. Toss the onion slices with the melted butter and transfer them to the air fryer basket. Air-fry at 400°F for 15 minutes, shaking the basket several times during the cooking process. Add the mushrooms and Worcestershire sauce to the onions and stir to combine. Air-fry at 400°F for an additional 10 minutes. Season with salt and freshly ground black pepper.
3. Lay two of the tortillas on a cutting board. Top each tortilla with ½ cup of the grated cheese, half of the onion and mushroom mixture and then finally another ½ cup of the cheese. Place the remaining tortillas on top of the cheese and press down firmly.
4. Brush the air fryer basket with a little oil. Place a quesadilla in the basket and brush the top with a little oil. Secure the top tortilla to the bottom with three toothpicks and air-fry at 400°F for 5 minutes. Flip the quesadilla over by inverting it onto a plate and sliding it back into the basket. Remove the toothpicks and brush the other side with oil. Air-fry for an additional 3 minutes.
5. Invert the quesadilla onto a cutting board and cut it into 4 or 6 triangles. Serve immediately.

Tacos

Servings: 24

Cooking Time: 8 Minutes Per Batch

Ingredients:

- 1 24-count package 4-inch corn tortillas
- 1½ cups refried beans (about ¾ of a 15-ounce can)
- 4 ounces sharp Cheddar cheese, grated
- ½ cup salsa
- oil for misting or cooking spray

Directions:

1. Preheat air fryer to 390°F.
2. Wrap refrigerated tortillas in damp paper towels and microwave for 30 to 60 seconds to warm. If necessary, rewarm tortillas as you go to keep them soft enough to fold without breaking.
3. Working with one tortilla at a time, top with 1 tablespoon of beans, 1 tablespoon of grated cheese, and 1 teaspoon of salsa. Fold over and press down very gently on the center. Press edges firmly all around to seal. Spray both sides with oil or cooking spray.
4. Cooking in two batches, place half the tacos in the air fryer basket. To cook 12 at a time, you may need to stand them upright and lean some against the sides of basket. It's okay if they're crowded as long as you leave a little room for air to circulate around them.
5. Cook for 8 minutes or until golden brown and crispy.
6. Repeat steps 4 and 5 to cook remaining tacos.

Broccoli Cheddar Stuffed Potatoes

Servings: 2

Cooking Time: 42 Minutes

Ingredients:

- 2 large russet potatoes, scrubbed
- 1 tablespoon olive oil
- salt and freshly ground black pepper
- 2 tablespoons butter
- ¼ cup sour cream
- 3 tablespoons half-and-half (or milk)
- 1¼ cups grated Cheddar cheese, divided
- ¾ teaspoon salt
- freshly ground black pepper
- 1 cup frozen baby broccoli florets, thawed and drained

Directions:

1. Preheat the air fryer to 400°F.
2. Rub the potatoes all over with olive oil and season generously with salt and freshly ground black pepper. Transfer the potatoes into the air fryer basket and air-fry for 30 minutes, turning the potatoes over halfway through the cooking process.
3. Remove the potatoes from the air fryer and let them rest for 5 minutes. Cut a large oval out of the top of both potatoes. Leaving half an inch of potato flesh around the edge of the potato, scoop the inside of the potato out and into a large bowl to prepare the potato filling. Mash the scooped potato filling with a fork and add the butter, sour cream, half-and-half, 1 cup of the grated Cheddar cheese, salt and pepper to taste. Mix well and then fold in the broccoli florets.
4. Stuff the hollowed out potato shells with the potato and broccoli mixture. Mound the filling high in the potatoes – you will have more filling than room in the potato shells.
5. Transfer the stuffed potatoes back to the air fryer basket and air-fry at 360°F for 10 minutes. Sprinkle the remaining Cheddar cheese on top of each stuffed potato, lower the heat to 330°F and air-fry for an additional minute or two to melt cheese.

Spicy Vegetable And Tofu Shake Fry

Servings: 4

Cooking Time: 17 Minutes

Ingredients:

- 4 teaspoons canola oil, divided
- 2 tablespoons rice wine vinegar
- 1 tablespoon sriracha chili sauce
- ¼ cup soy sauce*
- ½ teaspoon toasted sesame oil
- 1 teaspoon minced garlic
- 1 tablespoon minced fresh ginger
- 8 ounces extra firm tofu
- ½ cup vegetable stock or water
- 1 tablespoon honey
- 1 tablespoon cornstarch
- ½ red onion, chopped
- 1 red or yellow bell pepper, chopped
- 1 cup green beans, cut into 2-inch lengths
- 4 ounces mushrooms, sliced
- 2 scallions, sliced
- 2 tablespoons fresh cilantro leaves
- 2 teaspoons toasted sesame seeds

Directions:

1. Combine 1 tablespoon of the oil, vinegar, sriracha sauce, soy sauce, sesame oil, garlic and ginger in a small bowl. Cut the tofu into bite-sized cubes and toss the tofu in with the marinade while you prepare the other vegetables. When you are ready to start cooking, remove the tofu from the marinade and set it aside. Add the water, honey and cornstarch to the marinade and bring to a simmer on the stovetop, just until the sauce thickens. Set the sauce aside.
2. Preheat the air fryer to 400°F.
3. Toss the onion, pepper, green beans and mushrooms in a bowl with a little canola oil and season with salt. Air-fry at 400°F for 11 minutes, shaking the basket and tossing the vegetables every few minutes. When the vegetables are cooked to your preferred doneness, remove them from the air fryer and set aside.
4. Add the tofu to the air fryer basket and air-fry at 400°F for 6 minutes, shaking the basket a few times during the cooking process. Add the vegetables back to the basket and air-fry for another minute. Transfer the vegetables and tofu to a large bowl, add the scallions and cilantro leaves and toss with the sauce. Serve over rice with sesame seeds sprinkled on top.

Curried Potato, Cauliflower And Pea Turnovers

Servings: 4

Cooking Time: 40 Minutes

Ingredients:

- Dough:
- 2 cups all-purpose flour
- ½ teaspoon baking powder
- 1 teaspoon salt
- freshly ground black pepper
- ¼ teaspoon dried thyme
- ¼ cup canola oil
- ½ to ⅔ cup water
- Turnover Filling:
- 1 tablespoon canola or vegetable oil
- 1 onion, finely chopped
- 1 clove garlic, minced
- 1 tablespoon grated fresh ginger
- ½ teaspoon cumin seeds
- ½ teaspoon fennel seeds
- 1 teaspoon curry powder
- 2 russet potatoes, diced
- 2 cups cauliflower florets
- ½ cup frozen peas
- 2 tablespoons chopped fresh cilantro
- salt and freshly ground black pepper
- 2 tablespoons butter, melted
- mango chutney, for serving

Directions:

1. Start by making the dough. Combine the flour, baking powder, salt, pepper and dried thyme in a mixing bowl or the bowl of a stand mixer. Drizzle in the canola oil and pinch it together with your fingers to turn the flour into a crumby mixture. Stir in the water (enough to bring the dough together). Knead the dough for 5 minutes or so until it is smooth. Add a little more water or flour as needed. Let the dough rest while you make the turnover filling.
2. Preheat a large skillet on the stovetop over medium-high heat. Add the oil and sauté the onion until it starts to become tender – about 4 minutes. Add the garlic and ginger and continue to cook for another minute. Add the dried spices and toss everything to coat. Add the potatoes and cauliflower to the skillet and pour in 1½ cups of water. Simmer everything together for 20 to 25 minutes, or until the potatoes are soft and most of the water has evaporated. If the water has evaporated and the vegetables still need more time, just add a little water and continue to simmer until everything is tender. Stir well, crushing the potatoes and cauliflower a little as you do so. Stir in the peas and cilantro, season to taste with salt and freshly ground black pepper and set aside to cool.
3. Divide the dough into 4 balls. Roll the dough balls out into ¼-inch thick circles. Divide the cooled potato filling between the dough circles, placing a mound of the filling on one side of each piece of dough, leaving an empty border around the edge of the dough. Brush the edges of the dough with a

little water and fold one edge of circle over the filling to meet the other edge of the circle, creating a half moon. Pinch the edges together with your fingers and then press the edge with the tines of a fork to decorate and seal.

4. Preheat the air fryer to 380°F.
5. Spray or brush the air fryer basket with oil. Brush the turnovers with the melted butter and place 2 turnovers into the air fryer basket. Air-fry for 15 minutes. Flip the turnovers over and air-fry for another 5 minutes. Repeat with the remaining 2 turnovers.
6. These will be very hot when they come out of the air fryer. Let them cool for at least 20 minutes before serving warm with mango chutney.

Asparagus, Mushroom And Cheese Soufflés

Servings: 3

Cooking Time: 21 Minutes

Ingredients:

- butter
- grated Parmesan cheese
- 3 button mushrooms, thinly sliced
- 8 spears asparagus, sliced ½-inch long
- 1 teaspoon olive oil
- 1 tablespoon butter
- 4½ teaspoons flour
- pinch paprika
- pinch ground nutmeg
- salt and freshly ground black pepper
- ½ cup milk
- ½ cup grated Gruyère cheese or other Swiss cheese (about 2 ounces)
- 2 eggs, separated

Directions:

1. Butter three 6-ounce ramekins and dust with grated Parmesan cheese. (Butter the ramekins and then coat the butter with Parmesan by shaking it around in the ramekin and dumping out any excess.)
2. Preheat the air fryer to 400°F.
3. Toss the mushrooms and asparagus in a bowl with the olive oil. Transfer the vegetables to the air fryer and air-fry for 7 minutes, shaking the basket once or twice to redistribute the Ingredients while they cook.
4. While the vegetables are cooking, make the soufflé base. Melt the butter in a saucepan on the stovetop over medium heat. Add the flour, stir and cook for a minute or two. Add the paprika, nutmeg, salt and pepper. Whisk in the milk and bring the mixture to a simmer to thicken. Remove the pan from the heat and add the cheese, stirring to melt. Let the mixture cool for just a few minutes and then whisk the egg yolks in, one at a time. Stir in the cooked mushrooms and asparagus. Let this soufflé base cool.
5. In a separate bowl, whisk the egg whites to soft peak stage (the point at which the whites can almost stand up on the end of your whisk). Fold the whipped egg whites into the soufflé base, adding a little at a time.
6. Preheat the air fryer to 330°F.
7. Transfer the batter carefully to the buttered ramekins, leaving about ½-inch at the top. Place the ramekins into the air fryer basket and air-fry for 14 minutes. The soufflés should have risen nicely and be brown on top. Serve immediately.

Pizza Portobello Mushrooms

Servings: 2

Cooking Time: 18 Minutes

Ingredients:

- 2 portobello mushroom caps, gills removed (see Figure 13-1)
- 1 teaspoon extra-virgin olive oil
- ¼ cup diced onion
- 1 teaspoon minced garlic
- 1 medium zucchini, shredded
- 1 teaspoon dried oregano
- ½ teaspoon black pepper
- ¼ teaspoon salt
- ⅓ cup marinara sauce
- ¼ cup shredded part-skim mozzarella cheese
- ¼ teaspoon red pepper flakes
- 2 tablespoons Parmesan cheese
- 2 tablespoons chopped basil

Directions:

1. Preheat the air fryer to 370°F.
2. Lightly spray the mushrooms with an olive oil mist and place into the air fryer to cook for 10 minutes, cap side up.
3. Add the olive oil to a pan and sauté the onion and garlic together for about 2 to 4 minutes. Stir in the zucchini, oregano, pepper, and salt, and continue to cook. When the zucchini has cooked down (usually about 4 to 6 minutes), add in the marinara sauce. Remove from the heat and stir in the mozzarella cheese.
4. Remove the mushrooms from the air fryer basket when cooking completes. Reset the temperature to 350°F.
5. Using a spoon, carefully stuff the mushrooms with the zucchini marinara mixture.
6. Return the stuffed mushrooms to the air fryer basket and cook for 5 to 8 minutes, or until the cheese is lightly browned. You should be able to easily insert a fork into the mushrooms when they're cooked.
7. Remove the mushrooms and sprinkle the red pepper flakes, Parmesan cheese, and fresh basil over the top.
8. Serve warm.

Eggplant Parmesan

Servings: 4

Cooking Time: 8 Minutes Per Batch

Ingredients:

- 1 medium eggplant, 6–8 inches long
- salt
- 1 large egg
- 1 tablespoon water
- ⅔ cup panko breadcrumbs
- ⅓ cup grated Parmesan cheese, plus more for serving
- 1 tablespoon Italian seasoning
- ¾ teaspoon oregano
- oil for misting or cooking spray
- 1 24-ounce jar marinara sauce
- 8 ounces spaghetti, cooked
- pepper

Directions:

1. Preheat air fryer to 390°F.
2. Leaving peel intact, cut eggplant into 8 round slices about ¾-inch thick. Salt to taste.
3. Beat egg and water in a shallow dish.
4. In another shallow dish, combine panko, Parmesan, Italian seasoning, and oregano.
5. Dip eggplant slices in egg wash and then crumbs, pressing lightly to coat.
6. Mist slices with oil or cooking spray.
7. Place 4 eggplant slices in air fryer basket and cook for 8 minutes, until brown and crispy.
8. While eggplant is cooking, heat marinara sauce.
9. Repeat step 7 to cook remaining eggplant slices.
10. To serve, place cooked spaghetti on plates and top with marinara and eggplant slices. At the table, pass extra Parmesan cheese and freshly ground black pepper.

DESSERTS AND SWEETS

Blueberry Cheesecake Tartlets

Servings: 9

Cooking Time: 6 Minutes

Ingredients:

- 8 ounces cream cheese, softened
- ¼ cup sugar
- 1 egg
- ½ teaspoon vanilla extract
- zest of 2 lemons, divided
- 9 mini graham cracker tartlet shells*
- 2 cups blueberries
- ½ teaspoon ground cinnamon
- juice of ½ lemon
- ¼ cup apricot preserves

Directions:

1. Preheat the air fryer to 330°F.
2. Combine the cream cheese, sugar, egg, vanilla and the zest of one lemon in a medium bowl and blend until smooth by hand or with an electric hand mixer. Pour the cream cheese mixture into the tartlet shells.
3. Air-fry 3 tartlets at a time at 330°F for 6 minutes, rotating them in the air fryer basket halfway through the cooking time.
4. Combine the blueberries, cinnamon, zest of one lemon and juice of half a lemon in a bowl. Melt the apricot preserves in the microwave or over low heat in a saucepan. Pour the apricot preserves over the blueberries and gently toss to coat.
5. Allow the cheesecakes to cool completely and then top each one with some of the blueberry mixture. Garnish the tartlets with a little sugared lemon peel and refrigerate until you are ready to serve.

Puff Pastry Apples

Servings: 4

Cooking Time: 10 Minutes

Ingredients:

- 3 Rome or Gala apples, peeled
- 2 tablespoons sugar
- 1 teaspoon all-purpose flour
- 1 teaspoon ground cinnamon
- ⅛ teaspoon ground ginger
- pinch ground nutmeg
- 1 sheet puff pastry
- 1 tablespoon butter, cut into 4 pieces
- 1 egg, beaten
- vegetable oil
- vanilla ice cream (optional)
- caramel sauce (optional)

Directions:

1. Remove the core from the apple by cutting the four sides off the apple around the core. Slice the pieces of apple into thin half-moons, about ¼-inch thick. Combine the sugar, flour, cinnamon, ginger, and nutmeg in a large bowl. Add the apples to the bowl and gently toss until the apples are evenly coated with the spice mixture. Set aside.
2. Cut the puff pastry sheet into a 12-inch by 12-inch square. Then quarter the sheet into four 6-inch squares. Save any remaining pastry for decorating the apples at the end.
3. Divide the spiced apples between the four puff pastry squares, stacking the apples in the center of each square and placing them flat on top of each other in a circle. Top the apples with a piece of the butter.
4. Brush the four edges of the pastry with the egg wash. Bring the four corners of the pastry together, wrapping them around the apple slices and pinching them together at the top in the style of a "beggars purse" appetizer. Fold the ends of the pastry corners down onto the apple making them look like leaves. Brush the entire apple with the egg wash.
5. Using the leftover dough, make leaves to decorate the apples. Cut out 8 leaf shapes, about 1½-inches long, "drawing" the leaf veins on the pastry leaves with a paring knife. Place 2 leaves on the top of each apple, tucking the ends of the leaves under the pastry in the center of the apples. Brush the top of the leaves with additional egg wash. Sprinkle the entire apple with some granulated sugar.
6. Preheat the air fryer to 350°F.
7. Spray or brush the inside of the air fryer basket with oil. Place the apples in the basket and air-fry for 6 minutes. Carefully turn the apples over – it's easiest to remove one apple, then flip the others over and finally return the last apple to the air fryer. Air-fry for an additional 4 minutes.
8. Serve the puff pastry apples warm with vanilla ice cream and drizzle with some caramel sauce.

Oreo-coated Peanut Butter Cups

Servings:8

Cooking Time: 4 Minutes

Ingredients:

- 8 Standard ¾-ounce peanut butter cups, frozen
- ⅓ cup All-purpose flour
- 2 Large egg white(s), beaten until foamy
- 16 Oreos or other creme-filled chocolate sandwich cookies, ground to crumbs in a food processor
- Vegetable oil spray

Directions:

1. Set up and fill three shallow soup plates or small pie plates on your counter: one for the flour, one for the beaten egg white(s), and one for the cookie crumbs.
2. Dip a frozen peanut butter cup in the flour, turning it to coat all sides. Shake off any excess, then set it in the beaten egg white(s). Turn it to coat all sides, then let any excess egg white slip back into the rest. Set the candy bar in the cookie crumbs. Turn to coat on all parts, even the sides. Dip the peanut butter cup back in the egg white(s) as before, then into the cookie crumbs as before, making sure you have a solid, even coating all around the cup. Set aside while you dip and coat the remaining cups.
3. When all the peanut butter cups are dipped and coated, lightly coat them on all sides with the vegetable oil spray. Set them on a plate and freeze while the air fryer heats.
4. Preheat the air fryer to 400°F.
5. Set the dipped cups wider side up in the basket with as much air space between them as possible. Air-fry undisturbed for 4 minutes, or until they feel soft but the coating is set.
6. Turn off the machine and remove the basket from it. Set aside the basket with the fried cups for 10 minutes. Use a nonstick-safe spatula to transfer the fried cups to a wire rack. Cool for at least another 5 minutes before serving.

Maple Cinnamon Cheesecake

Servings: 4

Cooking Time: 12 Minutes

Ingredients:

- 6 sheets of cinnamon graham crackers
- 2 tablespoons butter
- 8 ounces Neufchâtel cream cheese
- 3 tablespoons pure maple syrup
- 1 large egg
- ½ teaspoon ground cinnamon
- ¼ teaspoon salt

Directions:

1. Preheat the air fryer to 350°F.
2. Place the graham crackers in a food processor and process until crushed into a flour. Mix with the butter and press into a mini air-fryer-safe pan lined at the bottom with parchment paper. Place in the air fryer and cook for 4 minutes.
3. In a large bowl, place the cream cheese and maple syrup. Use a hand mixer or stand mixer and beat together until smooth. Add in the egg, cinnamon, and salt and mix on medium speed until combined.
4. Remove the graham cracker crust from the air fryer and pour the batter into the pan.
5. Place the pan back in the air fryer, adjusting the temperature to 315°F. Cook for 18 minutes. Carefully remove when cooking completes. The top should be lightly browned and firm.
6. Keep the cheesecake in the pan and place in the refrigerator for 3 or more hours to firm up before serving.

Cherry Hand Pies

Servings: 8

Cooking Time: 8 Minutes

Ingredients:

- 4 cups frozen or canned pitted tart cherries (if using canned, drain and pat dry)
- 2 teaspoons lemon juice
- ½ cup sugar
- ¼ cup cornstarch
- 1 teaspoon vanilla extract
- 1 Basic Pie Dough (see the preceding recipe) or store-bought pie dough

Directions:

1. In a medium saucepan, place the cherries and lemon juice and cook over medium heat for 10 minutes, or until the cherries begin to break down.
2. In a small bowl, stir together the sugar and cornstarch. Pour the sugar mixture into the cherries, stirring constantly. Cook the cherry mixture over low heat for 2 to 3 minutes, or until thickened. Remove from the heat and stir in the vanilla extract. Allow the cherry mixture to cool to room temperature, about 30 minutes.
3. Meanwhile, bring the pie dough to room temperature. Divide the dough into 8 equal pieces. Roll out the dough to ¼-inch thickness in circles. Place ¼ cup filling in the center of each rolled dough. Fold the dough to create a half-circle. Using a fork, press around the edges to seal the hand pies. Pierce the top of the pie with a fork for steam release while cooking. Continue until 8 hand pies are formed.
4. Preheat the air fryer to 350°F.
5. Place a single layer of hand pies in the air fryer basket and spray with cooking spray. Cook for 8 to 10 minutes or until golden brown and cooked through.

Donut Holes

Servings: 13

Cooking Time: 12 Minutes

Ingredients:

- 6 tablespoons Granulated white sugar
- 1½ tablespoons Butter, melted and cooled
- 2 tablespoons (or 1 small egg, well beaten) Pasteurized egg substitute, such as Egg Beaters
- 6 tablespoons Regular or low-fat sour cream (not fat-free)
- ¾ teaspoon Vanilla extract
- 1⅔ cups All-purpose flour
- ¾ teaspoon Baking powder
- ¼ teaspoon Table salt
- Vegetable oil spray

Directions:

1. Preheat the air fryer to 350°F .
2. Whisk the sugar and melted butter in a medium bowl until well combined. Whisk in the egg substitute or egg , then the sour cream and vanilla until smooth. Remove the whisk and stir in the flour, baking powder, and salt with a wooden spoon just until a soft dough forms.
3. Use 2 tablespoons of this dough to create a ball between your clean palms. Set it aside and continue making balls: 8 more for the small batch, 12 more for the medium batch, or 17 more for the large one.
4. Coat the balls in the vegetable oil spray, then set them in the basket with as much air space between them as possible. Even a fraction of an inch will be enough, but they should not touch. Air-fry undisturbed for 12 minutes, or until browned and cooked through. A toothpick inserted into the center of a ball should come out clean.
5. Pour the contents of the basket onto a wire rack. Cool for at least 5 minutes before serving.

Giant Oatmeal–peanut Butter Cookie

Servings: 4

Cooking Time: 18 Minutes

Ingredients:

- 1 cup Rolled oats (not quick-cooking or steel-cut oats)
- ½ cup All-purpose flour
- ½ teaspoon Ground cinnamon
- ½ teaspoon Baking soda
- ⅓ cup Packed light brown sugar
- ¼ cup Solid vegetable shortening
- 2 tablespoons Natural-style creamy peanut butter
- 3 tablespoons Granulated white sugar
- 2 tablespoons (or 1 small egg, well beaten) Pasteurized egg substitute, such as Egg Beaters
- ⅓ cup Roasted, salted peanuts, chopped
- Baking spray

Directions:

1. Preheat the air fryer to 350°F .
2. Stir the oats, flour, cinnamon, and baking soda in a bowl until well combined.
3. Using an electric hand mixer at medium speed, beat the brown sugar, shortening, peanut butter, granulated white sugar, and egg substitute or egg (as applicable) until smooth and creamy, about 3 minutes, scraping down the inside of the bowl occasionally.
4. Scrape down and remove the beaters. Fold in the flour mixture and peanuts with a rubber spatula just until all the flour is moistened and the peanut bits are evenly distributed in the dough.
5. For a small air fryer, coat the inside of a 6-inch round cake pan with baking spray. For a medium air fryer, coat the inside of a 7-inch round cake pan with baking spray. And for a large air fryer, coat the inside of an 8-inch round cake pan with baking spray. Scrape and gently press the dough into the prepared pan, spreading it into an even layer to the perimeter.
6. Set the pan in the basket and air-fry undisturbed for 18 minutes, or until well browned.
7. Transfer the pan to a wire rack and cool for 15 minutes. Loosen the cookie from the perimeter with a spatula, then invert the pan onto a cutting board and let the cookie come free. Remove the pan and reinvert the cookie onto the wire rack. Cool for 5 minutes more before slicing into wedges to serve.

Custard

Servings: 4

Cooking Time: 45 Minutes

Ingredients:

- 2 cups whole milk
- 2 eggs
- ¼ cup sugar
- ⅛ teaspoon salt
- ¼ teaspoon vanilla
- cooking spray
- ⅛ teaspoon nutmeg

Directions:

1. In a blender, process milk, egg, sugar, salt, and vanilla until smooth.
2. Spray a 6 x 6-inch baking pan with nonstick spray and pour the custard into it.
3. Cook at 300°F for 45 minutes. Custard is done when the center sets.
4. Sprinkle top with the nutmeg.
5. Allow custard to cool slightly.
6. Serve it warm, at room temperature, or chilled.

Sea-salted Caramel Cookie Cups

Servings: 12

Cooking Time: 12 Minutes

Ingredients:

- ⅓ cup butter
- ¼ cup brown sugar
- 1 teaspoon vanilla extract
- 1 large egg
- 1 cup all-purpose flour
- ½ cup old-fashioned oats
- ½ teaspoon baking soda
- ¼ teaspoon salt
- ⅓ cup sea-salted caramel chips

Directions:

1. Preheat the air fryer to 300°F.
2. In a large bowl, cream the butter with the brown sugar and vanilla. Whisk in the egg and set aside.
3. In a separate bowl, mix the flour, oats, baking soda, and salt. Then gently mix the dry ingredients into the wet. Fold in the caramel chips.
4. Divide the batter into 12 silicon muffin liners. Place the cookie cups into the air fryer basket and cook for 12 minutes or until a toothpick inserted in the center comes out clean.
5. Remove and let cool 5 minutes before serving.

Blueberry Crisp

Servings: 6

Cooking Time: 13 Minutes

Ingredients:

- 3 cups Fresh or thawed frozen blueberries
- ⅓ cup Granulated white sugar
- 1 tablespoon Instant tapioca
- ⅓ cup All-purpose flour
- ⅓ cup Rolled oats (not quick-cooking or steel-cut)
- ⅓ cup Chopped walnuts or pecans
- ⅓ cup Packed light brown sugar
- 5 tablespoons plus 1 teaspoon (⅔ stick) Butter, melted and cooled
- ¾ teaspoon Ground cinnamon
- ¼ teaspoon Table salt

Directions:

1. Preheat the air fryer to 400°F.
2. Mix the blueberries, granulated white sugar, and instant tapioca in a 6-inch round cake pan for a small batch, a 7-inch round cake pan for a medium batch, or an 8-inch round cake pan for a large batch.
3. When the machine is at temperature, set the cake pan in the basket and air-fry undisturbed for 5 minutes, or just until the blueberries begin to bubble.
4. Meanwhile, mix the flour, oats, nuts, brown sugar, butter, cinnamon, and salt in a medium bowl until well combined.
5. When the blueberries have begun to bubble, crumble this flour mixture evenly on top. Continue air-frying undisturbed for 8 minutes, or until the topping has browned a bit and the filling is bubbling.
6. Use two hot pads or silicone baking mitts to transfer the cake pan to a wire rack. Cool for at least 10 minutes or to room temperature before serving.

S'mores Pockets

Servings: 6

Cooking Time: 5 Minutes

Ingredients:

- 12 sheets phyllo dough, thawed
- 1½ cups butter, melted
- ¾ cup graham cracker crumbs
- 1 (7-ounce) Giant Hershey's® milk chocolate bar
- 12 marshmallows, cut in half

Directions:

1. Place one sheet of the phyllo on a large cutting board. Keep the rest of the phyllo sheets covered with a slightly damp, clean kitchen towel. Brush the phyllo sheet generously with some melted butter. Place a second phyllo sheet on top of the first and brush it with more butter. Repeat with one more phyllo sheet until you have a stack of 3 phyllo sheets with butter brushed between the layers. Cover the phyllo sheets with one quarter of the graham cracker crumbs leaving a 1-inch border on one of the short ends of the rectangle. Cut the phyllo sheets lengthwise into 3 strips.
2. Take 2 of the strips and crisscross them to form a cross with the empty borders at the top and to the left. Place 2 of the chocolate rectangles in the center of the cross. Place 4 of the marshmallow halves on top of the chocolate. Now fold the pocket together by folding the bottom phyllo strip up over the chocolate and marshmallows. Then fold the right side over, then the top strip down and finally the left side over. Brush all the edges generously with melted butter to seal shut. Repeat with the next three sheets of phyllo, until all the sheets have been used. You will be able to make 2 pockets with every second batch because you will have an extra graham cracker crumb strip from the previous set of sheets.
3. Preheat the air fryer to 350°F.
4. Transfer 3 pockets at a time to the air fryer basket. Air-fry at 350°F for 4 to 5 minutes, until the phyllo dough is light brown in color. Flip the pockets over halfway through the cooking process. Repeat with the remaining 3 pockets.
5. Serve warm.

Sweet Potato Pie Rolls

Servings:3

Cooking Time: 8 Minutes

Ingredients:

- 6 Spring roll wrappers
- 1½ cups Canned yams in syrup, drained
- 2 tablespoons Light brown sugar
- ¼ teaspoon Ground cinnamon
- 1 Large egg(s), well beaten
- Vegetable oil spray

Directions:

1. Preheat the air fryer to 400°F.
2. Set a spring roll wrapper on a clean, dry work surface. Scoop up ¼ cup of the pulpy yams and set along one edge of the wrapper, leaving 2 inches on each side of the yams. Top the yams with about 1 teaspoon brown sugar and a pinch of ground cinnamon. Fold the sides of the wrapper perpendicular to the yam filling up and over the filling, partially covering it. Brush beaten egg(s) over the side of the wrapper farthest from the yam. Starting with the yam end, roll the wrapper closed, ending at the part with the beaten egg that you can press gently to seal. Lightly coat the roll on all sides with vegetable oil spray. Set it aside seam side down and continue filling, rolling, and spraying the remaining wrappers in the same way.
3. Set the rolls seam side down in the basket with as much air space between them as possible. Air-fry undisturbed for 8 minutes, or until crisp and golden brown.
4. Use a nonstick-safe spatula and perhaps kitchen tongs for balance to gently transfer the rolls to a wire rack. Cool for at least 5 minutes or up to 30 minutes before serving.

FISH AND SEAFOOD RECIPES

Bacon-wrapped Scallops

Servings: 4

Cooking Time: 8 Minutes

Ingredients:

- 16 large scallops
- 8 bacon strips
- ½ teaspoon black pepper
- ¼ teaspoon smoked paprika

Directions:

1. Pat the scallops dry with a paper towel. Slice each of the bacon strips in half. Wrap 1 bacon strip around 1 scallop and secure with a toothpick. Repeat with the remaining scallops. Season the scallops with pepper and paprika.
2. Preheat the air fryer to 350°F.
3. Place the bacon-wrapped scallops in the air fryer basket and cook for 4 minutes, shake the basket, cook another 3 minutes, shake the basket, and cook another 1 to 3 to minutes. When the bacon is crispy, the scallops should be cooked through and slightly firm, but not rubbery. Serve immediately.

Italian Tuna Roast

Servings: 8

Cooking Time: 21 Minutes

Ingredients:

- cooking spray
- 1 tablespoon Italian seasoning
- ⅛ teaspoon ground black pepper
- 1 tablespoon extra-light olive oil
- 1 teaspoon lemon juice
- 1 tuna loin (approximately 2 pounds, 3 to 4 inches thick, large enough to fill a 6 x 6-inch baking dish)

Directions:

1. Spray baking dish with cooking spray and place in air fryer basket. Preheat air fryer to 390°F.
2. Mix together the Italian seasoning, pepper, oil, and lemon juice.
3. Using a dull table knife or butter knife, pierce top of tuna about every half inch: Insert knife into top of tuna roast and pierce almost all the way to the bottom.
4. Spoon oil mixture into each of the holes and use the knife to push seasonings into the tuna as deeply as possible.
5. Spread any remaining oil mixture on all outer surfaces of tuna.
6. Place tuna roast in baking dish and cook at 390°F for 20 minutes. Check temperature with a meat thermometer. Cook for an additional 1 minutes or until temperature reaches 145°F.
7. Remove basket from fryer and let tuna sit in basket for 10minutes.

Stuffed Shrimp

Servings: 4

Cooking Time: 12 Minutes Per Batch

Ingredients:

- 16 tail-on shrimp, peeled and deveined (last tail section intact)
- ¾ cup crushed panko breadcrumbs
- oil for misting or cooking spray
- Stuffing
- 2 6-ounce cans lump crabmeat
- 2 tablespoons chopped shallots
- 2 tablespoons chopped green onions
- 2 tablespoons chopped celery
- 2 tablespoons chopped green bell pepper
- ½ cup crushed saltine crackers
- 1 teaspoon Old Bay Seasoning
- 1 teaspoon garlic powder
- ¼ teaspoon ground thyme
- 2 teaspoons dried parsley flakes
- 2 teaspoons fresh lemon juice
- 2 teaspoons Worcestershire sauce
- 1 egg, beaten

Directions:

1. Rinse shrimp. Remove tail section (shell) from 4 shrimp, discard, and chop the meat finely.
2. To prepare the remaining 12 shrimp, cut a deep slit down the back side so that the meat lies open flat. Do not cut all the way through.
3. Preheat air fryer to 360°F.
4. Place chopped shrimp in a large bowl with all of the stuffing ingredients and stir to combine.
5. Divide stuffing into 12 portions, about 2 tablespoons each.
6. Place one stuffing portion onto the back of each shrimp and form into a ball or oblong shape. Press firmly so that stuffing sticks together and adheres to shrimp.
7. Gently roll each stuffed shrimp in panko crumbs and mist with oil or cooking spray.
8. Place 6 shrimp in air fryer basket and cook at 360°F for 10minutes. Mist with oil or spray and cook 2 minutes longer or until stuffing cooks through inside and is crispy outside.
9. Repeat step 8 to cook remaining shrimp.

Tuna Nuggets In Hoisin Sauce

Servings: 4

Cooking Time: 7 Minutes

Ingredients:

- ½ cup hoisin sauce
- 2 tablespoons rice wine vinegar
- 2 teaspoons sesame oil
- 1 teaspoon garlic powder
- 2 teaspoons dried lemongrass
- ¼ teaspoon red pepper flakes
- ½ small onion, quartered and thinly sliced
- 8 ounces fresh tuna, cut into 1-inch cubes
- cooking spray
- 3 cups cooked jasmine rice

Directions:

1. Mix the hoisin sauce, vinegar, sesame oil, and seasonings together.
2. Stir in the onions and tuna nuggets.
3. Spray air fryer baking pan with nonstick spray and pour in tuna mixture.
4. Cook at 390°F for 3minutes. Stir gently.
5. Cook 2minutes and stir again, checking for doneness. Tuna should be barely cooked through, just beginning to flake and still very moist. If necessary, continue cooking and stirring in 1-minute intervals until done.
6. Serve warm over hot jasmine rice.

Five Spice Red Snapper With Green Onions And Orange Salsa

Servings: 2

Cooking Time: 8 Minutes

Ingredients:

- 2 oranges, peeled, segmented and chopped
- 1 tablespoon minced shallot
- 1 to 3 teaspoons minced red Jalapeño or Serrano pepper
- 1 tablespoon chopped fresh cilantro
- lime juice, to taste
- salt, to taste
- 2 (5- to 6-ounce) red snapper fillets
- ½ teaspoon Chinese five spice powder
- salt and freshly ground black pepper
- vegetable or olive oil, in a spray bottle
- 4 green onions, cut into 2-inch lengths

Directions:

1. Start by making the salsa. Cut the peel off the oranges, slicing around the oranges to expose the flesh. Segment the oranges by cutting in between the membranes of the orange. Chop the segments roughly and combine in a bowl with the shallot, Jalapeño or Serrano pepper, cilantro, lime juice and salt. Set the salsa aside.
2. Preheat the air fryer to 400°F.
3. Season the fish fillets with the five-spice powder, salt and freshly ground black pepper. Spray both sides of the fish fillets with oil. Toss the green onions with a little oil.
4. Transfer the fish to the air fryer basket and scatter the green onions around the fish. Air-fry at 400°F for 8 minutes.
5. Remove the fish from the air fryer, along with the fried green onions. Serve with white rice and a spoonful of the salsa on top.

Lemon-roasted Salmon Fillets

Servings:3

Cooking Time: 7 Minutes

Ingredients:

- 3 6-ounce skin-on salmon fillets
- Olive oil spray
- 9 Very thin lemon slices
- ¾ teaspoon Ground black pepper
- ¼ teaspoon Table salt

Directions:

1. Preheat the air fryer to 400°F.
2. Generously coat the skin of each of the fillets with olive oil spray. Set the fillets skin side down on your work surface. Place three overlapping lemon slices down the length of each salmon fillet. Sprinkle them with the pepper and salt. Coat lightly with olive oil spray.
3. Use a nonstick-safe spatula to transfer the fillets one by one to the basket, leaving as much air space between them as possible. Air-fry undisturbed for 7 minutes, or until cooked through.
4. Use a nonstick-safe spatula to transfer the fillets to serving plates. Cool for only a minute or two before serving.

Shrimp Teriyaki

Servings:10

Cooking Time: 6 Minutes

Ingredients:

- 1 tablespoon Regular or low-sodium soy sauce or gluten-free tamari sauce
- 1 tablespoon Mirin or a substitute (see here)
- 1 teaspoon Ginger juice (see the headnote)
- 10 Large shrimp (20–25 per pound), peeled and deveined
- ⅔ cup Plain panko bread crumbs (gluten-free, if a concern)
- 1 Large egg
- Vegetable oil spray

Directions:

1. Whisk the soy or tamari sauce, mirin, and ginger juice in an 8- or 9-inch square baking pan until uniform. Add the shrimp and toss well to coat. Cover and refrigerate for 1 hour, tossing the shrimp in the marinade at least twice.
2. Preheat the air fryer to 400°F.
3. Thread a marinated shrimp on a 4-inch bamboo skewer by inserting the pointy tip at the small end of the shrimp, then guiding the skewer along the shrimp so that the tip comes out the thick end and the shrimp is flat along the length of the skewer. Repeat with the remaining shrimp. (You'll need eight 4-inch skewers for the small batch, 10 skewers for the medium batch, and 12 for the large.)
4. Pour the bread crumbs onto a dinner plate. Whisk the egg in the baking pan with any marinade that stayed behind. Lay the skewers in the pan, in as close to a single layer as possible. Turn repeatedly to make sure the shrimp is coated in the egg mixture.
5. One at a time, take a skewered shrimp out of the pan and set it in the bread crumbs, turning several times and pressing gently until the shrimp is evenly coated on all sides. Coat the shrimp with vegetable oil spray and set the skewer aside. Repeat with the remainder of the shrimp.
6. Set the skewered shrimp in the basket in one layer. Air-fry undisturbed for 6 minutes, or until pink and firm.
7. Transfer the skewers to a wire rack. Cool for only a minute or two before serving.

Shrimp "scampi"

Servings:4

Cooking Time: 5 Minutes

Ingredients:

- 1½ pounds Large shrimp (20–25 per pound), peeled and deveined
- ¼ cup Olive oil
- 2 tablespoons Minced garlic
- 1 teaspoon Dried oregano
- Up to 1 teaspoon Red pepper flakes
- ½ teaspoon Table salt
- 2 tablespoons White balsamic vinegar (see here)

Directions:

1. Preheat the air fryer to 400°F.
2. Stir the shrimp, olive oil, garlic, oregano, red pepper flakes, and salt in a large bowl until the shrimp are well coated.
3. When the machine is at temperature, transfer the shrimp to the basket. They will overlap and even sit on top of each other. Air-fry for 5 minutes, tossing and rearranging the shrimp twice to make sure the covered surfaces are exposed, until pink and firm.
4. Pour the contents of the basket into a serving bowl. Pour the vinegar over the shrimp while hot and toss to coat.

Shrimp Patties

Servings: 4

Cooking Time: 10 Minutes

Ingredients:

- ½ pound shelled and deveined raw shrimp
- ¼ cup chopped red bell pepper
- ¼ cup chopped green onion
- ¼ cup chopped celery
- 2 cups cooked sushi rice
- ½ teaspoon garlic powder
- ½ teaspoon Old Bay Seasoning
- ½ teaspoon salt
- 2 teaspoons Worcestershire sauce
- ½ cup plain breadcrumbs
- oil for misting or cooking spray

Directions:

1. Finely chop the shrimp. You can do this in a food processor, but it takes only a few pulses. Be careful not to overprocess into mush.
2. Place shrimp in a large bowl and add all other ingredients except the breadcrumbs and oil. Stir until well combined.
3. Preheat air fryer to 390°F.
4. Shape shrimp mixture into 8 patties, no more than ½-inch thick. Roll patties in breadcrumbs and mist with oil or cooking spray.
5. Place 4 shrimp patties in air fryer basket and cook at 390°F for 10 minutes, until shrimp cooks through and outside is crispy.
6. Repeat step 5 to cook remaining shrimp patties.

Salmon Puttanesca En Papillotte With Zucchini

Servings: 2

Cooking Time: 17 Minutes

Ingredients:

- 1 small zucchini, sliced into ¼-inch thick half moons
- 1 teaspoon olive oil
- salt and freshly ground black pepper
- 2 (5-ounce) salmon fillets
- 1 beefsteak tomato, chopped (about 1 cup)
- 1 tablespoon capers, rinsed
- 10 black olives, pitted and sliced
- 2 tablespoons dry vermouth or white wine 2 tablespoons butter
- ¼ cup chopped fresh basil, chopped

Directions:

1. Preheat the air fryer to 400°F.
2. Toss the zucchini with the olive oil, salt and freshly ground black pepper. Transfer the zucchini into the air fryer basket and air-fry for 5 minutes, shaking the basket once or twice during the cooking process.
3. Cut out 2 large rectangles of parchment paper – about 13-inches by 15-inches each. Divide the air-fried zucchini between the two pieces of parchment paper, placing the vegetables in the center of each rectangle.
4. Place a fillet of salmon on each pile of zucchini. Season the fish very well with salt and pepper. Toss the tomato, capers, olives and vermouth (or white wine) together in a bowl. Divide the tomato mixture between the two fish packages, placing it on top of the fish fillets and pouring any juice out of the bowl onto the fish. Top each fillet with a tablespoon of butter.
5. Fold up each parchment square. Bring two edges together and fold them over a few times, leaving some space above the fish. Twist the open sides together and upwards so they can serve as handles for the packet, but don't let them extend beyond the top of the air fryer basket.
6. Place the two packages into the air fryer and air-fry at 400°F for 12 minutes. The packages should be puffed up and slightly browned when fully cooked. Once cooked, let the fish sit in the parchment for 2 minutes.
7. Serve the fish in the parchment paper, or if desired, remove the parchment paper before serving. Garnish with a little fresh basil.

SANDWICHES AND BURGERS RECIPES

Sausage And Pepper Heros

Servings: 3

Cooking Time: 11 Minutes

Ingredients:

- 3 links (about 9 ounces total) Sweet Italian sausages (gluten-free, if a concern)
- 1½ Medium red or green bell pepper(s), stemmed, cored, and cut into ½-inch-wide strips
- 1 medium Yellow or white onion(s), peeled, halved, and sliced into thin half-moons
- 3 Long soft rolls, such as hero, hoagie, or Italian sub rolls (gluten-free, if a concern), split open lengthwise
- For garnishing Balsamic vinegar
- For garnishing Fresh basil leaves

Directions:

1. Preheat the air fryer to 400°F.
2. When the machine is at temperature, set the sausage links in the basket in one layer and air-fry undisturbed for 5 minutes.
3. Add the pepper strips and onions. Continue air-frying, tossing and rearranging everything about once every minute, for 5 minutes, or until the sausages are browned and an instant-read meat thermometer inserted into one of the links registers 160°F.
4. Use a nonstick-safe spatula and kitchen tongs to transfer the sausages and vegetables to a cutting board. Set the rolls cut side down in the basket in one layer (working in batches as necessary) and air-fry undisturbed for 1 minute, to toast the rolls a bit and warm them up. Set 1 sausage with some pepper strips and onions in each warm roll, sprinkle balsamic vinegar over the sandwich fillings, and garnish with basil leaves.

Best-ever Roast Beef Sandwiches

Servings: 6

Cooking Time: 30-50 Minutes

Ingredients:

- 2½ teaspoons Olive oil
- 1½ teaspoons Dried oregano
- 1½ teaspoons Dried thyme
- 1½ teaspoons Onion powder
- 1½ teaspoons Table salt
- 1½ teaspoons Ground black pepper
- 3 pounds Beef eye of round
- 6 Round soft rolls, such as Kaiser rolls or hamburger buns (gluten-free, if a concern), split open lengthwise
- ¾ cup Regular, low-fat, or fat-free mayonnaise (gluten-free, if a concern)
- 6 Romaine lettuce leaves, rinsed
- 6 Round tomato slices (¼ inch thick)

Directions:

1. Preheat the air fryer to 350°F .
2. Mix the oil, oregano, thyme, onion powder, salt, and pepper in a small bowl. Spread this mixture all over the eye of round.
3. When the machine is at temperature, set the beef in the basket and air-fry for 30 to 50 minutes (the range depends on the size of the cut), turning the meat twice, until an instant-read meat thermometer inserted into the thickest piece of the meat registers 130°F for rare, 140°F for medium, or 150°F for well-done.
4. Use kitchen tongs to transfer the beef to a cutting board. Cool for 10 minutes. If serving now, carve into ⅛-inch-thick slices. Spread each roll with 2 tablespoons mayonnaise and divide the beef slices between the rolls. Top with a lettuce leaf and a tomato slice and serve. Or set the beef in a container, cover, and refrigerate for up to 3 days to make cold roast beef sandwiches anytime.

Chili Cheese Dogs

Servings: 3

Cooking Time: 12 Minutes

Ingredients:

- ¾ pound Lean ground beef
- 1½ tablespoons Chile powder
- 1 cup plus 2 tablespoons Jarred sofrito
- 3 Hot dogs (gluten-free, if a concern)
- 3 Hot dog buns (gluten-free, if a concern), split open lengthwise
- 3 tablespoons Finely chopped scallion
- 9 tablespoons (a little more than 2 ounces) Shredded Cheddar cheese

Directions:

1. Crumble the ground beef into a medium or large saucepan set over medium heat. Brown well, stirring often to break up the clumps. Add the chile powder and cook for 30 seconds, stirring the whole time. Stir in the sofrito and bring to a simmer. Reduce the heat to low and simmer, stirring occasionally, for 5 minutes. Keep warm.
2. Preheat the air fryer to 400°F.
3. When the machine is at temperature, put the hot dogs in the basket and air-fry undisturbed for 10 minutes, or until the hot dogs are bubbling and blistered, even a little crisp.
4. Use kitchen tongs to put the hot dogs in the buns. Top each with a ½ cup of the ground beef mixture, 1 tablespoon of the minced scallion, and 3 tablespoons of the cheese. (The scallion should go under the cheese so it superheats and wilts a bit.) Set the filled hot dog buns in the basket and air-fry undisturbed for 2 minutes, or until the cheese has melted.
5. Remove the basket from the machine. Cool the chili cheese dogs in the basket for 5 minutes before serving.

Perfect Burgers

Servings: 3

Cooking Time: 13 Minutes

Ingredients:

- 1 pound 2 ounces 90% lean ground beef
- 1½ tablespoons Worcestershire sauce (gluten-free, if a concern)
- ½ teaspoon Ground black pepper
- 3 Hamburger buns (gluten-free if a concern), split open

Directions:

1. Preheat the air fryer to 375°F .
2. Gently mix the ground beef, Worcestershire sauce, and pepper in a bowl until well combined but preserving as much of the meat's fibers as possible. Divide this mixture into two 5-inch patties for the small batch, three 5-inch patties for the medium, or four 5-inch patties for the large. Make a thumbprint indentation in the center of each patty, about halfway through the meat.
3. Set the patties in the basket in one layer with some space between them. Air-fry undisturbed for 10 minutes, or until an instant-read meat thermometer inserted into the center of a burger registers 160°F (a medium-well burger). You may need to add 2 minutes cooking time if the air fryer is at 360°F.
4. Use a nonstick-safe spatula, and perhaps a flatware fork for balance, to transfer the burgers to a cutting board. Set the buns cut side down in the basket in one layer (working in batches as necessary) and air-fry undisturbed for 1 minute, to toast a bit and warm up. Serve the burgers in the warm buns.

Thai-style Pork Sliders

Servings: 4

Cooking Time: 15 Minutes

Ingredients:

- 11 ounces Ground pork
- 2½ tablespoons Very thinly sliced scallions, white and green parts
- 4 teaspoons Minced peeled fresh ginger
- 2½ teaspoons Fish sauce (gluten-free, if a concern)
- 2 teaspoons Thai curry paste (see the headnote; gluten-free, if a concern)
- 2 teaspoons Light brown sugar
- ¾ teaspoon Ground black pepper
- 4 Slider buns (gluten-free, if a concern)

Directions:

1. Preheat the air fryer to 375°F .
2. Gently mix the pork, scallions, ginger, fish sauce, curry paste, brown sugar, and black pepper in a bowl until well combined. With clean, wet hands, form about ⅓ cup of the pork mixture into a slider about 2½ inches in diameter. Repeat until you use up all the meat—3 sliders for the small batch, 4 for the medium, and 6 for the large. (Keep wetting your hands to help the patties adhere.)
3. When the machine is at temperature, set the sliders in the basket in one layer. Air-fry undisturbed for 14 minutes, or until the sliders are golden brown and caramelized at their edges and an instant-read meat thermometer inserted into the center of a slider registers 160°F.
4. Use a nonstick-safe spatula, and perhaps a flatware fork for balance, to transfer the sliders to a cutting board. Set the buns cut side down in the basket in one layer (working in batches as necessary) and air-fry undisturbed for 1 minute, to toast a bit and warm up. Serve the sliders warm in the buns.

Crunchy Falafel Balls

Servings: 8

Cooking Time: 16 Minutes

Ingredients:

- 2½ cups Drained and rinsed canned chickpeas
- ¼ cup Olive oil
- 3 tablespoons All-purpose flour
- 1½ teaspoons Dried oregano
- 1½ teaspoons Dried sage leaves
- 1½ teaspoons Dried thyme
- ¾ teaspoon Table salt
- Olive oil spray

Directions:

1. Preheat the air fryer to 400°F.
2. Place the chickpeas, olive oil, flour, oregano, sage, thyme, and salt in a food processor. Cover and process into a paste, stopping the machine at least once to scrape down the inside of the canister.
3. Scrape down and remove the blade. Using clean, wet hands, form 2 tablespoons of the paste into a ball, then continue making 9 more balls for a small batch, 15 more for a medium one, and 19 more for a large batch. Generously coat the balls in olive oil spray.
4. Set the balls in the basket in one layer with a little space between them and air-fry undisturbed for 16 minutes, or until well browned and crisp.
5. Dump the contents of the basket onto a wire rack. Cool for 5 minutes before serving.

Lamb Burgers

Servings: 3

Cooking Time: 17 Minutes

Ingredients:

- 1 pound 2 ounces Ground lamb
- 3 tablespoons Crumbled feta
- 1 teaspoon Minced garlic
- 1 teaspoon Tomato paste
- ¾ teaspoon Ground coriander
- ¾ teaspoon Ground dried ginger
- Up to ⅛ teaspoon Cayenne
- Up to a ⅛ teaspoon Table salt (optional)
- 3 Kaiser rolls or hamburger buns (gluten-free, if a concern), split open

Directions:

1. Preheat the air fryer to 375°F .
2. Gently mix the ground lamb, feta, garlic, tomato paste, coriander, ginger, cayenne, and salt (if using) in a bowl until well combined, trying to keep the bits of cheese intact. Form this mixture into two 5-inch patties for the small batch, three 5-inch patties for the medium, or four 5-inch patties for the large.
3. Set the patties in the basket in one layer and air-fry undisturbed for 16 minutes, or until an instant-read meat thermometer inserted into one burger registers 160°F. (The cheese is not an issue with the temperature probe in this recipe as it was for the Inside-Out Cheeseburgers, because the feta is so well mixed into the ground meat.)
4. Use a nonstick-safe spatula, and perhaps a flatware fork for balance, to transfer the burgers to a cutting board. Set the buns cut side down in the basket in one layer (working in batches as necessary) and air-fry undisturbed for 1 minute, to toast a bit and warm up. Serve the burgers warm in the buns.

Thanksgiving Turkey Sandwiches

Servings: 3

Cooking Time: 10 Minutes

Ingredients:

- 1½ cups Herb-seasoned stuffing mix (not cornbread-style; gluten-free, if a concern)
- 1 Large egg white(s)
- 2 tablespoons Water
- 3 5- to 6-ounce turkey breast cutlets
- Vegetable oil spray
- 4½ tablespoons Purchased cranberry sauce, preferably whole berry
- ⅛ teaspoon Ground cinnamon
- ⅛ teaspoon Ground dried ginger
- 4½ tablespoons Regular, low-fat, or fat-free mayonnaise (gluten-free, if a concern)
- 6 tablespoons Shredded Brussels sprouts
- 3 Kaiser rolls (gluten-free, if a concern), split open

Directions:

1. Preheat the air fryer to 375°F .
2. Put the stuffing mix in a heavy zip-closed bag, seal it, lay it flat on your counter, and roll a rolling pin over the bag to crush the stuffing mix to the consistency of rough sand. (Or you can pulse the stuffing mix to the desired consistency in a food processor.)
3. Set up and fill two shallow soup plates or small pie plates on your counter: one for the egg white(s), whisked with the water until foamy; and one for the ground stuffing mix.
4. Dip a cutlet in the egg white mixture, coating both sides and letting any excess egg white slip back into the rest. Set the cutlet in the ground stuffing mix and coat it evenly on both sides, pressing gently to coat well on both sides. Lightly coat the cutlet on both sides with vegetable oil spray, set it aside, and continue dipping and coating the remaining cutlets in the same way.
5. Set the cutlets in the basket and air-fry undisturbed for 10 minutes, or until crisp and brown. Use kitchen tongs to transfer the cutlets to a wire rack to cool for a few minutes.
6. Meanwhile, stir the cranberry sauce with the cinnamon and ginger in a small bowl. Mix the shredded Brussels sprouts and mayonnaise in a second bowl until the vegetable is evenly coated.
7. Build the sandwiches by spreading about 1½ tablespoons of the cranberry mixture on the cut side of the bottom half of each roll. Set a cutlet on top, then spread about 3 tablespoons of the Brussels sprouts mixture evenly over the cutlet. Set the other half of the roll on top and serve warm.

Chicken Spiedies

Servings: 3

Cooking Time: 12 Minutes

Ingredients:

- 1¼ pounds Boneless skinless chicken thighs, trimmed of any fat blobs and cut into 2-inch pieces
- 3 tablespoons Red wine vinegar
- 2 tablespoons Olive oil
- 2 tablespoons Minced fresh mint leaves
- 2 tablespoons Minced fresh parsley leaves
- 2 teaspoons Minced fresh dill fronds
- ¾ teaspoon Fennel seeds
- ¾ teaspoon Table salt
- Up to a ¼ teaspoon Red pepper flakes
- 3 Long soft rolls, such as hero, hoagie, or Italian sub rolls (gluten-free, if a concern), split open lengthwise
- 4½ tablespoons Regular or low-fat mayonnaise (not fat-free; gluten-free, if a concern)
- 1½ tablespoons Distilled white vinegar
- 1½ teaspoons Ground black pepper

Directions:

1. Mix the chicken, vinegar, oil, mint, parsley, dill, fennel seeds, salt, and red pepper flakes in a zip-closed plastic bag. Seal, gently massage the marinade ingredients into the meat, and refrigerate for at least 2 hours or up to 6 hours. (Longer than that and the meat can turn rubbery.)
2. Set the plastic bag out on the counter (to make the contents a little less frigid). Preheat the air fryer to 400°F.
3. When the machine is at temperature, use kitchen tongs to set the chicken thighs in the basket (discard any remaining marinade) and air-fry undisturbed for 6 minutes. Turn the thighs over and continue air-frying undisturbed for 6 minutes more, until well browned, cooked through, and even a little crunchy.
4. Dump the contents of the basket onto a wire rack and cool for 2 or 3 minutes. Divide the chicken evenly between the rolls. Whisk the mayonnaise, vinegar, and black pepper in a small bowl until smooth. Drizzle this sauce over the chicken pieces in the rolls.

Lightning Source UK Ltd.
Milton Keynes UK
UKHW051300181122
412426UK00021B/210

9 781802 448962